Crying In Silence

Crying In Silence

Shelley Lynn O'Leary

Library of Congress Control Number: 2012900235
ISBN: Hardcover   978-1-4691-4640-9
                 Softcover   978-1-4691-4639-3
                 Ebook   978-1-4691-4641-6

This book was printed in the United States of America.

To order additional copies of this book, contact:
Xlibris Corporation
1-888-795-4274
www.Xlibris.com
Orders@Xlibris.com
110484

For my Mother, who has always been there for me whenever a need arose. Without her wonderful guidance and caring attitude, I would not have the self-confidence that I have today. Her love for me has been a constant theme as she attempted to nurture my total development and appreciation for the life that I have been given. She is my God-given gift.

FOREWARD

I AM WRITING THIS book to share my life experience to date so that others who may be afflicted with a like disability may find some solace in knowing that they are not alone. Having gown up in a Title IX era that was largely ignored by public schools and the general public, I was oblivious to the benefits that should have been provided to me and others as children. I thank those who came forward to serve as our ambassadors to provide the rightful treatment and care that we deserved. My Mother was one of those individuals who negated every obstacle in her path to ensure that my needs were properly cared for under the Law. Her dedication to succeed in any and all endeavors proved to be decisive, not only for myself, but for many others in our local school district. This book is, therefore, dedicated to her.

THE INTENSITY OF DESPERATION

I HAVE THE FEELING of immobility, as one might sense impending doom when trapped in a burning building. I'm not feeling quite right! Fighting my fear, I am unable to shake the thought that there is nothing I can do. I begin to feel that my body is going through something major. Something is definitely wrong, and that I'm in danger! However, I don't know why! There is a 'weight' on my chest, holding me down, as I experience a feeling of falling backward onto my back in my bed. I sense that there is someone sitting on me and weighing 'a ton of bricks'. In addition, I can't do anything about it.

I try to move my arms and legs, but I'm not able! Panic sets in. I start worrying about my personal safety! I begin 'seizing' seconds later. *"Oh, God, please do not let me fall out of bed!"* I'm thinking that if I fall over the side, I'll hit my head because I won't be able to break my fall. My head is in a terrible and confusing state of fog-oriented stupor. In addition, my body is at the mercy of this horrible paralysis. My mind wills my body to stop, but my body simply ignores my mind! I can't control what's going on!

My little brother Timmy is sleeping in the next bed. I am seven years old and he is five. I don't want him to see me this way. *Please God, don't let him wake up and see his older Sister in this inescapable and trapped experience!"*

My Father comes into the bedroom and sees me convulsing. He is kneeling beside my bed trying to tell me that it's going to be all right. I try to move my eyes to look at him, but they do not move. Dad, there's something wrong, but the words don't come right! I can't talk to him! *"Dad, please help me!"* my mind pleads. Why won't my body stop shaking this way? What is happening to me? I am so frightened and scared to death. My mind tells me, though, that my Parents are here and that it's going to be O.K.

Dad makes sure that I don't fall out of bed and hit my head on the floor. Next, Mom comes into the room and she is panicking! *"What's going on?"* I ask my Father. I cannot even talk to them to try to let them know what I'm thinking. My body is jerking and there is nothing I can do to stop it.

"Lynn, she is having a seizure. Get to the phone and call for 'Rescue' to get over there right away!" My parents have never seen me this way before.

I see my Father hovering over me and telling me that it's going to be O.K. *"Dad"*, I try to say, *"It's not O.K.! Please do something to make this stop!"* Timmy is still sleeping! Oh, God, someone please make this all go away!

Five minutes later, I'm told the Gorham Rescue vehicle arrives at our house. Thank you, God, for having the Town Rescue right across the street from where we live. A young paramedic, who wants to become an EMT someday, and an elderly paramedic come into the bedroom. I'm still convulsing. The older EMT looks down at me and smiles. "Shelley," he says calmly, "You're going to be alright, Honey. We're going to get you some help." Mom is hysterical! Dad is trying to comfort my Mother.

SHELLEY LYNN O'LEARY

They take me downstairs and to the ambulance. God, I can't fall off this stretcher! I'm still in my nightgown with the Smurf characters on it. What if someone in the neighborhood sees me with only my nightgown on! Mom gets into the ambulance with me and the paramedic. Dad is in his car and is going to follow the ambulance to the hospital. My older brother Michael who was sleeping in the same room as Timmy and me has been told to take care of his younger brother while we're gone. Mike is concerned for me. He's 17 years old and I look up to him. He tells me before I leave the house that everything is going to be O.K. I believe him. I see the kind paramedic comforting Mom, hugging her, and telling her not to worry.

In the ambulance, I'm given something in my arm. The needle they stick into me stings, but it stops my convulsing after several minutes. I don't know how long I've been in this uncontrollable physical state. However, I've stop shaking. Moreover, I am tired. I am *so very tired*! I could sleep for a year, if I had to! What did I just go through?

Mom is still crying beside me. I want to tell her that it's O.K. now, Mom!

I'm going to be alright. I am so very tired! In addition, I fall asleep before the ambulance arrives at the hospital. Much later, I wake up and see my older brother Mike at my beside. His girlfriend is there beside him. I'm glad to see them both.

This was my first experience with a *'grand-mal'* seizure. It happened because of my cerebral palsy, instigated by the lack of oxygen to my brain at the moment of my birth. No one knows exactly why this happened to me, although there is conjecture. Later, it was determined that my Mother's blood pressure had dropped dramatically in the operating room just prior to my coming into this world, via caesarian section. It was believed that there was a shortened period of time when my brain was 'starved' from receiving oxygen, resulting in specific brain area tissue being compromised. My parents are eventually told that I have approximately 10% brain tissue that is deadened. My Epilepsy results when the electrical impulses are conveyed via brain synapses in the "live" portion that attempt to bridge with synapses in the "dead" 10% area. The result is a "short circuit" that my body essentially rejects and subsequently rebels by throwing me into a "seizure state".

SHELLEY AND TIMMY DURING
THE EARLY SEIZURE YEARS

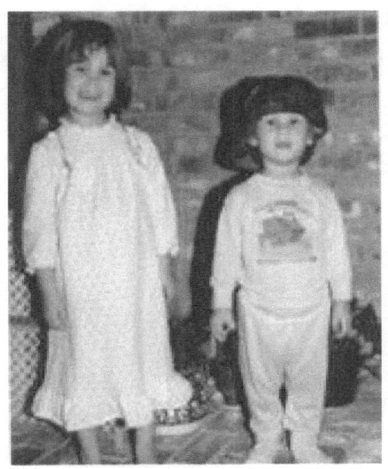

M Y FATHER, WHO was present during the birth process, remarked later that I had come into this world with eyes 'wide open' and in seeming distress. It was the only way he could describe it. The operating room nurses and the attending doctor delivering me had the appearance of concern. I was immediately given to an attending nurse in the 'OR' and 'cleaned up'.

My Mother was wheeled back to her hospital room. She asked to see me. The nurse brought me in and gave me to my Mother, who smiled at her second born, a healthy girl, or so she thought. My Father had been led out of the operating room and told that he could be with Mom and me shortly. Dad took the brief opportunity to call his parents in Louisiana to let them know that they had a new granddaughter. Everyone was happy.

During the course of the ensuing six months following my birth, my Father began to notice a lack of mobility in my arm and leg on my left side. When I would swing my leg(s) up and down, my right leg would move, but not my left. My parents also noted that my left hand would ball up in a fist and that, when touched, or manipulated to open, there was difficulty in keeping the hand pliable. Both my parents developed major concerns that there appeared to be a non-use issue with my left hand and left leg. This prompted an appointment with a Neurologist, a Doctor Walter Allan, in Portland, Maine.

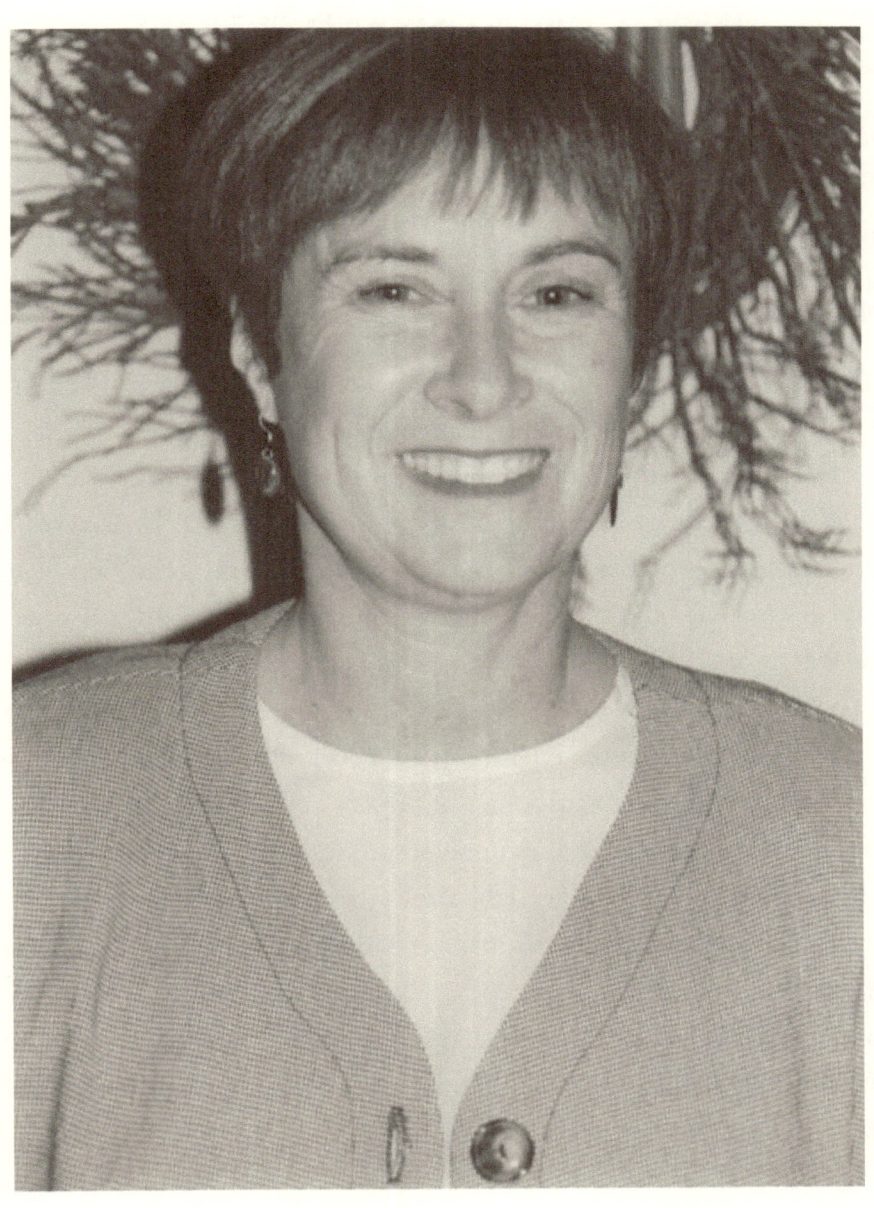

MY MOTHER

INITIAL DIAGNOSIS AND THERAPY

F OLLOWING MY INITIAL meeting with the neurologist, my Mother was devastated. My Father later told me that she was quite distraught at finding out that her Daughter had cerebral palsy. Dad tried to comfort her by saying that life could have been worse for Shelley, or not at all. What my Father was trying to tell my Mother was that I was alive and that Dr. Allan, even though he told my Parents that my condition would never improve for the better, neither would it ever worsen. It was what it was for the remainder of my life.

This was small consolation for Mom. I believe she felt guilty at believing that she had been the cause for my physical disability. Had something been done to mitigate the drop in blood pressure that day in the operating room, I might not have suffered the stroke that caused the permanent brain damage. My Mom actually felt that she had some measure of control over what took place that October 31, 1979. She could not have been more wrong. It wasn't her control to take; it was the medical authority by her side that day that could have prevented the occurrence, as was later seen with the birth of my younger Brother Timmy.

In any event, it was what it was. Dr. Allan's seemingly brusque manner in giving the initial news to my Parents was only surface in nature, as Mom and Dad later learned over the course of my visits with him. Dr.

Allan became my medical Champion. Even though I treated him with an 'attitude' to his face, it was never personal. I treated every 'stranger' with an attitude. Even my immediate family 'suffered' from my behavior. I firmly believed and was convinced that, for some reason, my attitude, even as a young child, was directed toward life itself. In addition, in an ironic way, this "attitude" would toughen me when faced with life's everyday challenges. I believe God put me in my physical situation to be an eventual role model for others who suffered from similar debilitating conditions.

My cerebral palsy and seizure condition had begun their medical journey that day in Dr. Walter Allan's Park Avenue, Portland office. My Parents knew that I would not be the physically 'normal' second child in their Family. However, I know that they didn't truly care about that because they always showed how much they loved me in thought and deed. Little did I know then how very blessed I was to be surrounded with love and the respect for whom I was, rather than for whom I was not.

I have to admit that my relationship with Dr. Allan started in a "stormy" sort of way. I was sassy, and he was understanding; I was non-approachable, and he was understanding; I was obstinate, and he was understanding; I was reluctant to "give him the time of day", and he was understanding; I acted uncooperative, and he was understanding. If I could have given him "the finger", he would have been understanding. I simply could not wear this man down! In addition, I was a mature three year old!

Thus began my "love affair" with Dr. Allan's inability to turn me away. My parents later told me that, with all of my attempts to sabotage our relationship, it seemed to spur Dr. Allan on to love me even more for the "spunky" girl that I was.

I believe Dr. Allan saw my being rambunctious as a strength, an ability to deal with life's problems and not be overwhelmed by them. He also was perceptive in envisioning somehow my willingness to give back to the world a desire to show that I would not be deterred from helping others. He viewed me as someone who would empathize with others by assisting them to overcome their fear of existing as someone less than whole and less than "normal". Moreover, that this physical "less than normal" self-perception was perfectly alright in a world where challenges were there to be overcome.

My continued and frequent appointments with Dr. Allan were a Godsend to me. Every time we met, I tried my best to alienate him with my attitude, which seemed to spur on more deeply his affection for me. He seemed to thrive on my apparent disdainful treatment of him.

I know today that Dr. Walter Allan understood that my direction toward life's apparent "unfairness" would serve me well for the remainder of my life. In addition, I also believe that he was the only person to see my "thrust of the middle finger" at anything and everyone in life as my "protection measure" to withstand what cruelty I would face later on in the world. He couldn't have been more right about what I was all about.

Even though Dr. Walter Allan ceased being my Neurologist due to his leaving active practice in pursuit of research study in neurology, he remained a huge part in my life. After our absence from seeing one another for years, our meeting would "light up" his eyes as he remembered who I had been, and the young woman I had become.

SHELLEY LYNN O'LEARY

SHRINER'S HOSPITAL

MY GRANDFATHER, MY Mother's Father, was a key business Member and Officer serving on the Board of Directors for the Portland Civic Center. His local influence was wide reaching as a very successful John Hancock Insurance Agent in Northeastern Maine. As a result, he had cultivated some key contacts with the Shriner's Organization in Portland. Pap, as I referred to him, suggested to my Parents that I receive care at the Hospital located in Springfield, Massachusetts. My Parents agreed that it would certainly help me in establishing a base line for therapy and subsequent care in that regard.

After contact was made with the appropriate officials, I was granted an initial appointment as a three-year old to see a Specialist in the area of Cerebral Palsy. Springfield, Massachusetts was a three-hour drive from our home in Gorham, Maine. My younger brother Timmy had a rough time making the entire trip without becoming "fussy" in his car seat beside me. Nevertheless, we always seemed to make it without too much of a problem.

One of the best things about making this trip was that we were able to stay in a Motel for the night. Timmy and I slept in the same double bed beside Mom and Dad's. Before going to sleep, I "coerced" my parents into raiding the Motel vending machines for snacks while we watched television for the evening. Moreover, we could eat on the bed!

The next morning, there was always what they called a "continental" breakfast, whatever that meant. However, what was more important was what they had to eat! There were donuts and pastries, cereal, toast, and different juices. I think I was in Breakfast Heaven!

The first visit to Shriner's Hospital, Mom and Dad checked me in and we were asked to wait in a large room with a lot of parents and children, many with cerebral palsy. Not too long after sitting down, two or three CLOWNS, like in a circus, came into the waiting room and started talking to the boys and girls there. I had been sleeping on Dad's shoulder. I opened up my eyes and a clown's face was very close to mine! I have to admit that seeing them so tall and with all of the CLOWN makeup on really frightened me! One of them had got real close to me and I cringed and sought out Mom! My left arm and hand were really affected by this. I would raise my left arm and bend it at the elbow with my fist very tightly clenched! This would eventually become a signature posture whenever I truly felt very uneasy about a person or situation before me.

From that time, I was afraid of people made up to be a clown. With subsequent visits to Shriner's, Mom and Dad made sure that we were seated in an area with minimum chance for a Clown to come over to me. Even as a teen, my recollection of the many visits to Springfield, Massachusetts and to Shriner's would raise an uncomfortable memory of a frightening figure walking toward me with a face that was "scary" to me.

Although my visits began with a waiting period in a large community room, the doctors who saw me were very professional and helpful to my Parents. After only one visit when the Doctor asked me to walk back and forth in a hallway for his evaluation, he recommended that I wear a supportive device in my left shoe to assist in controlling the left foot "turning

SHELLEY LYNN O'LEARY

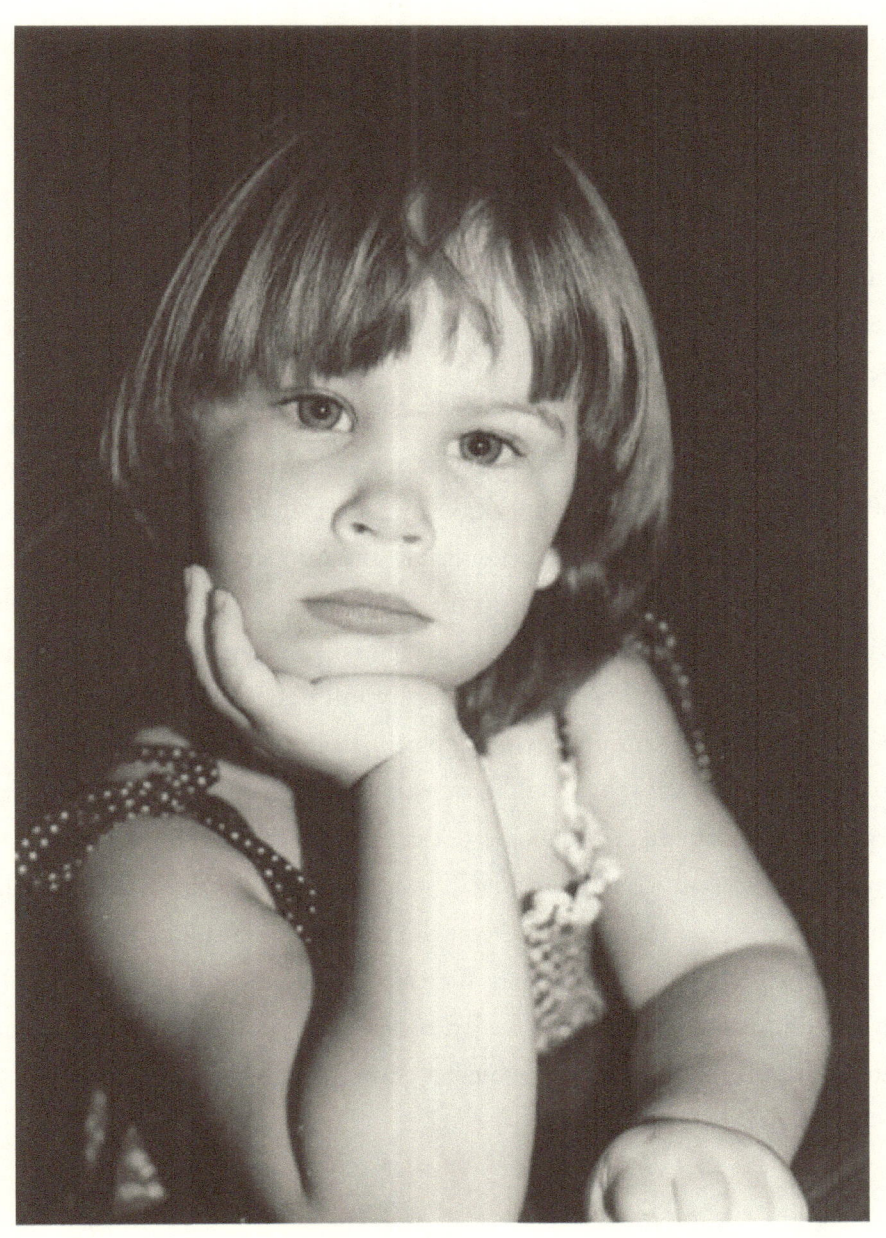

SHELLEY DURING SHRINER YEARS

in" excessively. To this day, I still wear the supportive device that has been a significant assist in allowing me to walk in a manner that produced less stress anatomically. However, I don't feel "normal" when I wear them.

Overall, we visited the Shriner's Hospital in Springfield for a little over two years. As Timmy and I were older each time, the trips to Springfield and to the Hospital represented an opportunity to sleep in a Motel with a vending machine and "Continental" breakfasts that seemed to get better an better each time we visited!

Overall, my Grandfather Pap was truly instrumental in getting me off "on the left foot", so to speak, with expert diagnosis and subsequent treatment that was extremely beneficial for many years to the present time. He wasn't the only one to take up the challenge to protect me and others with like physical disadvantages. There are many individuals in my life who have supported me in my development physically and psychologically. Each person provided me the opportunity to utilize my God-given inner strength to overcome obstacles that could have easily overcome my desire to grow as a person. The old adage that God doesn't present trials before us if we are unable to succeed was alive and well. It appears that, to this day, I am still "being pushed" to succeed by others who care for my physical and spiritual development. The following section deals with the most significant people in my life: those who never gave up on me and prompted me to pursue dreams that I may never have achieved without their total support.

SHELLEY LYNN O'LEARY

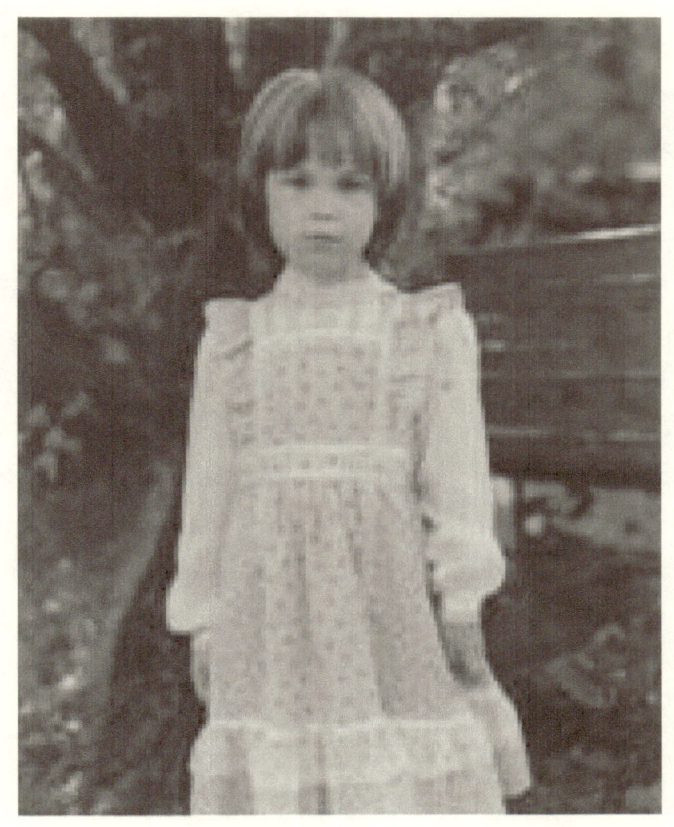

SHELLEY IN ELEMENTARY SCHOOL

MY LIFELONG CHAMPIONS

MY **MOTHER**: PERHAPS the single-most influential person is my life has been Mom. Together with her loving support during my learning days in elementary, and high school, and more importantly, my college years, my Mother was always there for me. I can never remember a single time when my Mother wasn't there sitting beside me and helping me understand my homework, or listening patiently to my social problems, both in and out of school. She truly taught me "how to learn!" She stressed that it was more important to accept that my learning would be comparatively more difficult than those without a physical disadvantage. Acceptance was the first step in recognizing that my learning would be difficult. Once I made a "pact" with myself that whatever I could do to gain information toward acquiring a learning methodology, a method that would work for me, I was on my way toward accepting my cognitive disability. I knew then that I would have to stop comparing myself to others in terms of how I gained knowledge. My "way" would have to be the "Best Way"!

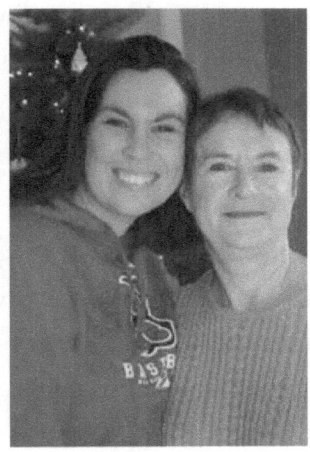

My Mother taught me how to ride a bike. This was a labor of love for my Mother because it actually took me a little over two years to master balance on the bicycle. When I would fall, she would encourage me to try again. Eventually, I would be able to ride comfortably, thereby eliciting praise from her. In addition, it was this praise that assisted me in knowing that there wasn't anything I couldn't do if I tried hard enough because my Mother would always be there to support me in every way.

She was patient in teaching me how to use my left hand in tying my shoes. There were times when I would become frustrated and tell myself that I just couldn't do it. My Mother wouldn't take that for an answer and would continue to encourage me in saying that such things were possible. She would "nudge" me to try again. Moreover, when I succeeded, there was a wonderful feeling of accomplishment!

It was this feeling of success after a "thousand" times of trying that spurned me on to develop a sense of reaching out and take a chance at completing a task, any task. My Mother's constant praise and recognition for what I had done served as a motivation for me to continue "to take the plunge" and not be afraid to try anything. In all of life's challenges, I was encouraged to be successful, even if it meant hard and arduous repetition. My Mother's message to me was to never give up. In addition, my constant reminder of my engrained motto of "My do it! "would always serve me well in anything I challenged myself in life.

In elementary school, my Mother was the very first person in Gorham to pick up the staff and be the standard-bearer for the physically disadvantaged in protecting the rights of students. My Mother got involved with the Gorham Elementary School after she saw injustices and total apathy directed toward those individuals whose rights were being violated in concert with the dictates of Title IX Law.

My physical therapy was conducted on the floor in the bathroom. When classroom "portables" were put out and located to the rear of the school, there was no provision for restroom accessibility for the disabled. The physically-challenged children at the school were ignored as we were left to fend for ourselves with no consideration given to our disabilities. There were no "ramps" for the wheel-chair borne students.

My Mother approached the school principal and informed her of my Mother's concerns. When action was not forthcoming to provide the Title IX services that were mandated by Law, she went to the School Board. It was only after she threatened to bring awareness of the Town of Gorham's shortcomings to the Maine Department of Education when she approached one of Maine's United States House of Representatives and it was then that something was eventually done to "push" local officials to "get off the dime" and start thinking about the physically disabled in a more positive light. It was a time for the physically-challenged to stop being regarded as "second-class citizens."

SHELLEY LYNN O'LEARY

As my Mother was adamant about not only protecting my own well-being, but those of all students at the then elementary school level, a group of concerned parents began to get together and asked my Mother to chair the group and be the spokesperson for its committee. There were scheduled meetings when parents would cite the frustrations they were experiencing because their child was being ignored or prejudiced against due to the physical disability. Issues like these served to fuel the fire in my Mother's heart that would not let the school "off the hook" for failing to adhere to the established educational mandates after the Congressmen had become involved in support of the parents' fight for justice. It didn't take long for the school to understand that to fight against a Federal Law would not serve it very well and that it was time to get its "house" in order before the appropriate agency forced it to do so, at the expense of their own employment.

Even though my Mother feels guilty for my disability occurring, she was always supportive of me by always being there when I needed her to be. With my schoolwork, my Mother helped me to learn in a way that made sense to me. My stroke at birth caused brain damage that affected the analytical side of my learning. Consequently, trying to "get" math was like learning a foreign language in one night. My Mother found ways to overcome this deficiency by appealing to common sense as an avenue for learning.

Memorization was also difficult for me. My Mother was also there to suggest different cues that, again, made sense to me and allowed me to be able to retain information, not only for exams, but for the rest of my life.

My writing skills were deficient and they showed in my inability to relay thoughts to a reader on paper. However, with constant practice, I eventually got to a point where I was able to feel more comfortable in my writing "skin".

An interesting anecdote about my Mother in having me initiate my own school papers has always brought a smile to our faces. When I needed to begin writing a term paper and I looked to my Mother to help me get it

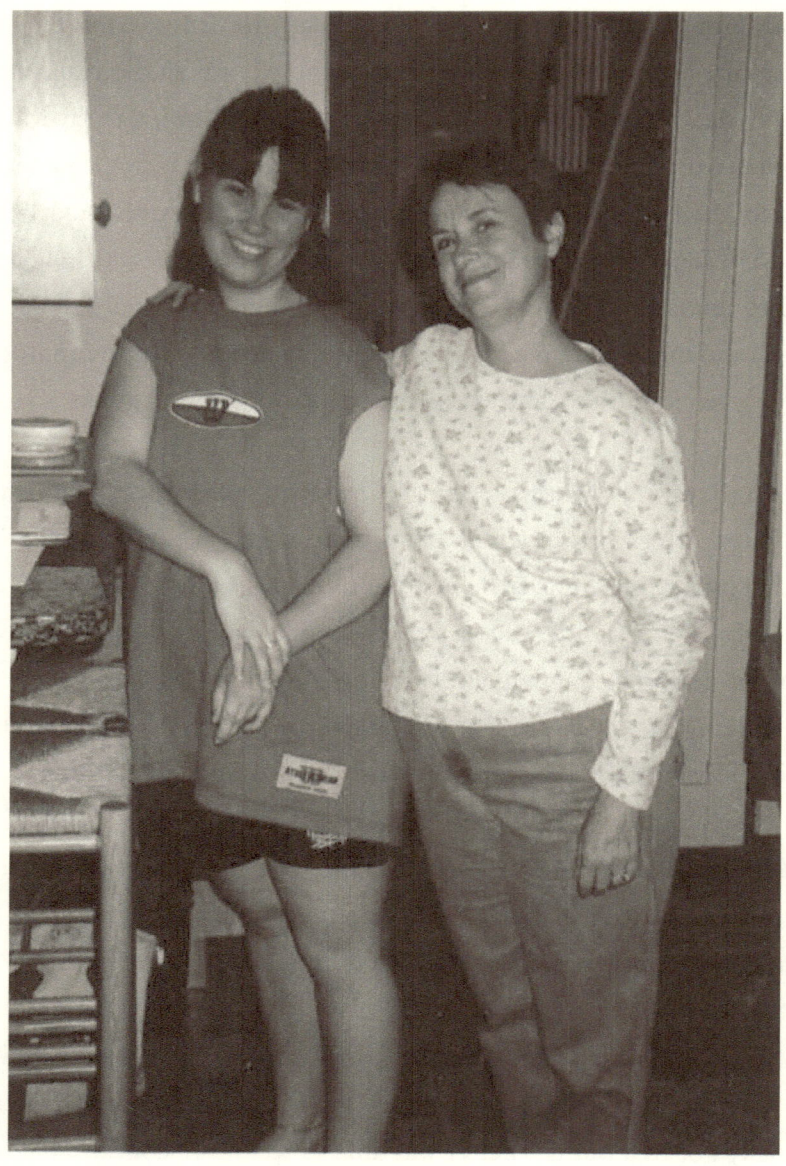

SHELLEY AND LYNN

SHELLEY LYNN O'LEARY

going, she would tell me that she needed to go outside and do just a little work in her garden. After two hours of waiting, I decided that, if I didn't get started, it would never get off the ground! Therefore, I would begin writing the paper on my own. When Mom would come in, I would have a lot of it done. This was her way of telling me that she had more confidence in me to complete a written project on my own and that she was really not needed as a "crutch" to realize I could achieve success on my own!

My Mother has taught me the value of helping others to cope with their own "afflictions" by having me recognize my own. As I seek confirmation that my disability is the work of a "Higher Power" at work, I use it to empathize and assist others to reach the same conclusion that I have about their own affliction so that they, in turn, may help others one day. It's akin to the movie, "Pay It Forward", a giving of oneself unselfishly so that others may learn to focus outward, rather than to dwell on their own personal inward.

MY FATHER: I was born on Halloween 1979. My Mother developed complications during the birth and I was subsequently deprived of oxygen. As a result, I incurred a mild form of cerebral palsy that affected my left side. I was able to walk, but with a pronounced slap in my step. My left arm and hand were more severely hampered and I used my hand more as an assist than for normal functional use. I also suffered from seizures due to the deadening of brain tissue incurred during birth.

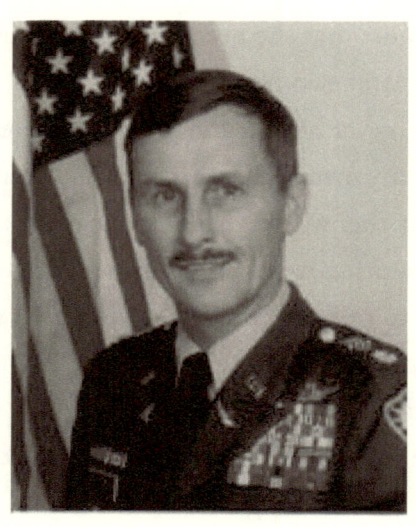

MY FATHER
LIEUTENANT COLONEL TIMOTHY J. O'LEARY, III

I honestly believe that I and my Mother's subsequent dealing with these physical abnormalities made both of us stronger. I, to this day, have "the heart of a lion", according to my Father. I have the spunk that is immeasurable in terms of 'never tell me that I can't do that!' At one point in a high school class, I showed my fellow students how to tie their shoes with one hand. There is nothing that I won't attempt. My motto was, *'My Do It!'*

When I was two years old, I was a climber. I would get on the furniture and with a pacifier in my mouth climb up onto our living room sofa and proceed to get to its highest point. When told to get down, I responded with silent defiance. In a restaurant I would stand in our booth and stare intently at the people eating their food. My look to others was one of a quest for daring someone to say something so I could let them know that I was not taking 'them prisoners' that day. I loved to be controversial, especially with my older brother Michael.

SHELLEY LYNN O'LEARY

One day, I walked over to Michael as he was trying to complete a homework assignment on the coffee table. I would quietly put my arm on the resource Michael was using to complete his assignment and then stare him down. When my brother told me to stop what I was doing, I kept my arm right were it was and merely continued to look at him with what was construed as, *'how dare you tell me what to do! I'll slap you into next Wednesday, Big Brother!'*

I had developed a not-so-unique answer to life's challenges by mastering the 'middle finger approach' to all events and people who stood in my way! Do I take after my Father?

I was making a 'show and tell' presentation to my elementary school classmates one day and my subject involved my older brother Michael. Because Michael was olive-skinned from Italian heritage, I proceeded to inform my classmates that Michael was my 'Black' brother. I don't really know if Michael realized this revelation! I am convinced he truly believes himself to be Caucasian though.

I earned two Associates' Degrees, one in Business Management, and the other in Therapeutic Recreation. All of this occurred after I was placed in a special education environment in high school. My determination to succeed in all endeavors surfaced following high school graduation. I found myself having a passion for helping others to succeed. In my work at the cerebral palsy center, I seem to have the God-given gift to assist children who need the care and love that help them to grow. I have worked with children diagnosed with autism.

"Other adults cannot accomplish what she can when willingly striving to earn the trust of an autistic child. They seem to flock to her as they sense they can rely on her to provide loving direction. She has an uncanny instinct about understanding the other person's affliction and his/her need to accept the caring that she can provide. All children love her; all children rely on her; and, all children view her as a surrogate parent who gently directs their lives in a positive and understanding manner," my Father said.

My Father goes on generously to say, "I firmly believe that she will earn and wear the title of Director one day. That day will be a glorious one for all children who will be cared for with understanding love. She is a Gift from God and, I feel, HE is extremely pleased with what HE is seeing. For Jesus said, 'Suffer the little children unto me.' She epitomes this directive, and there is no 'suffering' on her part in attempting to meet the needs of others. Helping others is engrained in her, just as a patchwork quilt is a work of beauty. Her soul is full of love for others. We were blessed when she came into this world, and this world is a much better place with her in it!"

My Father was proud that, due to my disability and the elementary school not providing the necessary concerns and care, in accordance with the Federal Title IX directive, my Mother picked up and raised the standard of discontent as high as she could. Mom was instrumental in providing for me and other disadvantaged students through her advocating for those requirements dictated by Title IX. My Mother got a support group together in the attempt to effect change, rightful change, for all deserving utmost consideration in accordance with the federal mandate. She worked tirelessly to make the facilities accessible by bringing legislative "heavy hitters" into the support group fold. Mom today is recognized as the one significant parent who successfully advocated for her child, and for all children in the Gorham School System. She was not to be denied in this very important quest for federal law compliance.

SHELLEY LYNN O'LEARY

My Dad goes on to say, "Shelley and I cross swords with one another every once in a while, but I wouldn't trade her for any other daughter. I fondly refer to my this day as 'My Favorite Daughter!' Of course, her feisty response is always, *'Yea, Dad, I'm your only Daughter!'* I wouldn't want another because she's the best that God could have blessed me with! As she works with the physically disabled, God's gift to her *is* her disability because she is able to give selflessly to others afflicted with what is considered as less than normal abilities to deal with life's challenges. Her Mentors are Dr. Allan, her Neurologist, and a lady who has been close to her for so many of my formative years, Susan Cody-Butler, her school Occupational Therapist whom she calls her Friend. These two have been very important mosaic pieces in her life because they have molded her to become a self-reliant, responsible, and a very accountable individual.

"She understand the needs of those children who love and adore her, children who need someone with whom they can share the joy in life that she innately provides lovingly and willingly. Her strength is in her past. In school she was shunned because of her disability. She was mocked and even attacked by other high students because she was 'different'. She didn't tell them about her epilepsy because she didn't know what would happen to her in the way of affecting her safety.

"One day she was negotiating a set of stairs coming from a class when a student reached out with her foot and purposely tripped her. Her books went flying as she fell to the floor. She picked herself up and, in a mature and classy manner, walked away as those bullying students laughed and engaged in self-congratulatory remarks that smacked of gross immaturity.

"These types of events have served her well! What I mean by this is that she is a firm believer that life's challenges and rewards even out in the end. With every negative thing that she has had to deal with in her life, her reward will be a most deserved and immense addition to this world and to Heaven's role."

My Father's alcoholism has always been a huge concern for me. When he would drink, he became a different person. My Father would become confrontational at the "drop of a hat". He wasn't physically mean, but he was non-approachable. One could tell when he had been drinking because the least conversation would often turn into a major issue with him. I despised what alcohol did to him. I loved my Father, but not the Alcoholic.

On one summertime afternoon, he had been drinking. He and I both knew this. After cutting the lawn at our home, he decided to get into his car and drive off. I presumed that he wanted to go to the store to buy additional beer.

I confronted him with his ability to drive in his inebriated state. My Dad insisted in getting into his car. I told him that if he did, I would call the police. My Father drove anyway. I called the police.

He was pulled over about a mile from our home. The police officer administered a sobriety test and he failed. My Father was then handcuffed and taken to the County jail. He was booked and incarcerated for eight hours. After bail was provided by my Mother at 2:30 in the morning, he was released into her care. My mother loved my Father and, despite her inner sense to leave him in jail to teach him "a lesson", she yielded, submitted bail, and drove him home.

My Dad was charged with DUI. His attorney plea-bargained it down to a Class D misdemeanor, driving-to-endanger. The end result was still the same: he had driven off in an inebriated state. He had broken the law. He lost his license for 90 days. Everyone who heard of this incident applauded my actions.

The end-result for my Father was a memory that he will never shake from his mind. There were indirect and lasting ensuing penalties for his actions over and above the 90-day license suspension. He was not able to acquire any subsequent employment relating to driving for a Company, in any capacity. My Father had been a helicopter pilot. As a consequence to his actions relating to the driving-to-endanger charge, his attempt to acquire a bona fide FAA Class II medical certificate was scrutinized adversely. Moreover, my Father loved flying. These were issues that he never held against me for my actions. He knew that I operated in "good faith" and in "protecting" others on the road that afternoon. I know that I did the right thing. Others praised me for taking the courage to do what I did. My Father, I believe, understands this, despite the actions on his part that caused him to self-inflict a nail in the coffin of never being able to fly again. My Dad is a proud person. He will never forget what happened that afternoon; he will never forgive himself for putting me in the position I took.

DR. WALTER ALLAN: This man was like an angel to me. I always felt safe with his care. When I would see him walk into my waiting room, I would instinctively relax. Everything was going to be alright when I saw him for an appointment. Dr. Allan understood me, as opposed to other neurologists whom I have seen to date. His departure from practice to go on to complete research in the field of neurology was my "loss" at the time. However, his research is sure to be a huge benefit to those many hundreds of individuals who will reap the benefit of his successful investigation into understanding and overcoming the malevolence of epilepsy.

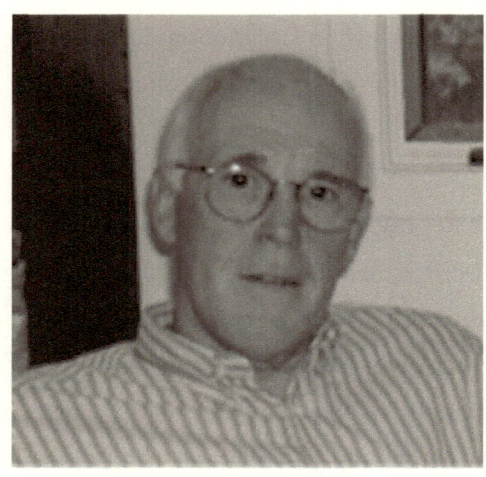

DR. WALTER ALLAN, NEUROLOGIST

SUSAN CODY-BUTLER: A truly outstanding Professional who helped me in so many ways to learn to live with my disability. Susan was my Occupational Therapist in my school system who worked with me in a most positive way. She is one of my "Angels" in life who provided me with the support and positive feedback that allowed me to understand that my physical limitations were only as severe as I myself made them out to be.

Susan allowed me to achieve success; I disavowed the word "failure". In providing me the confidence that I could accomplish my goals, albeit through hard work, I learned that life's restrictions are almost always arbitrarily placed upon ourselves. In addition, our successes result from a positive outlook in everything we try to do. My Mother and Susan worked extensively together to assist me to become the person I am today.

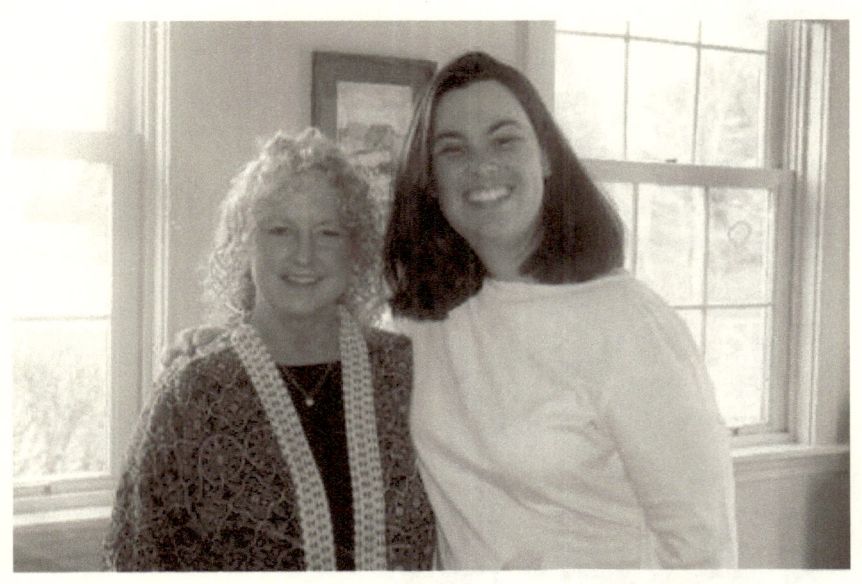

SUSAN CODY-BUTLER AND SHELLEY

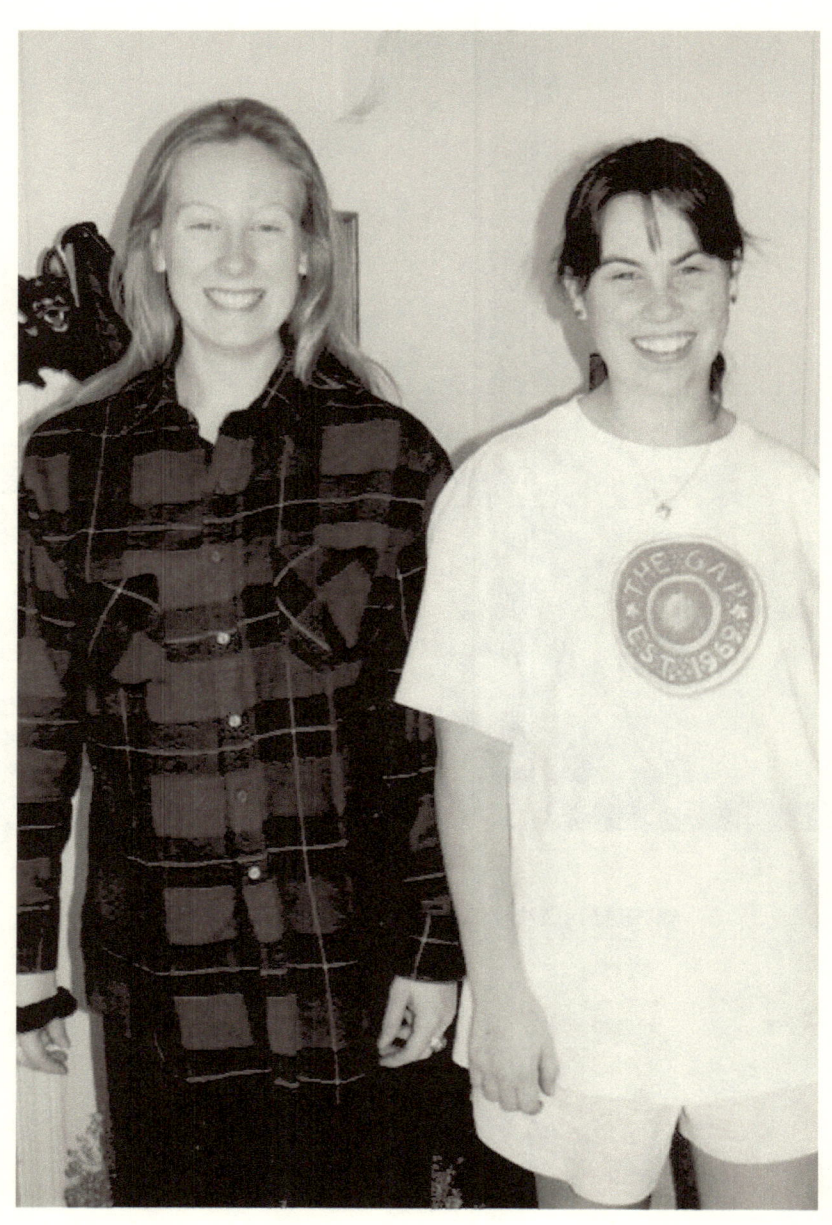

CRYSTAL AND SHELLEY

CRYSTAL CRANSTON: A Friend and Model of support for over 19 years. Crystal has been my Protector in High School and beyond. She never once gave up on me. As others would mock me, Crystal always treated me with the utmost of respect. We have spent some wonderful and memorable times together to include going on cruises to the Mediterranean as well as many other short trips to various locations in the State of Maine. She can very well attest to our enjoyment of the local ice cream establishment called "Sweets 'n Eats" in the summers. Where she was always there for me, I did my very best to support Crystal in any manner possible. This was especially true when she gave birth to Mariah during our Junior year at Gorham High school. I helped her get through those traumatic times when she had to deal with Family and the father of Mariah. When she did not have anyone to turn to, I wanted to be there for her. If there was ever a 'soul-mate friend", it is most certainly Crystal.

There was a time when I felt my life was not worth living. I told this to Crystal one day. Her response was something I needed to get me to stop with my self-pity and to accept the person that I truly was. At that moment, I felt that she was the only person outside of my Parents who truly cared about me. Her genuine friendship shined through and helped me to overcome my deep feeling of inferiority and lack of worth. She brought me back down to earth to face the true person that I was that day. I can honestly say that her comments helped me to face life honestly in that I was able to face forward in life as opposed to dwelling on the past that created my situation for the remainder of my existence.

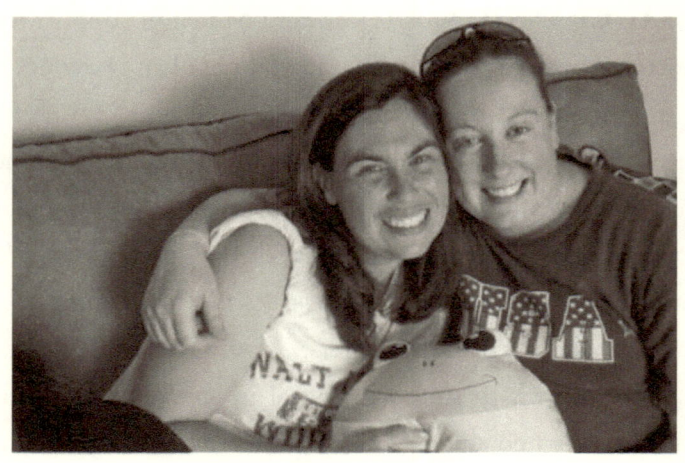

SHELLEY AND CRYSTAL

HUNTER KING: "Uncle" Hunter is like a second Father to me. He has a wonderful sense of humor and constantly keeps me "on my toes" with his one-liners! I believe he has also been one to find my "feistiness" attractive and endearing, as he himself is one known not to "take prisoners". He and I have always been a lot alike in that we both have always felt a strong need "to tell it like it is"! Hunter King has been in my life since birth. My Father and I will periodically make a luncheon date with him and use this as an opportunity to catch up with what has been going on in our lives. Dad and he coached Little League together for a number of years, and I know my Father has the greatest amount of respect for his willingness to give freely to others in need. "Uncle Hunter" constantly teases me that I would always look my "best" wearing only the "black and white" garb so commonly provided to the Sisters of "No-Mercy"! My first serious boyfriend will be in for a rude awakening when having to be grilled, not only by my Father and two Brothers, but by "Uncle" Hunter as well. I feel that his "vote of approval" will be the most—deciding vote of all!

SHELLEY LYNN O'LEARY

He was always kind and understanding. His friendly banter was always well-received. Every time we had the occasion to get together, he enriched my life significantly!

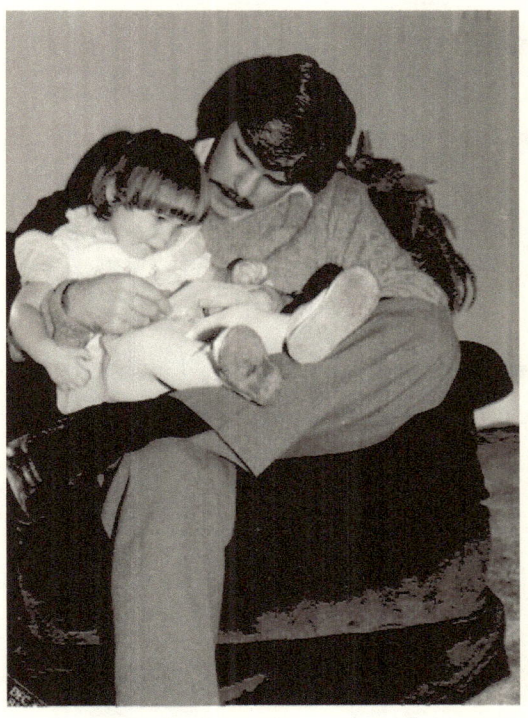

MARIAH CRANSTON: The Daughter to Crystal Cranston is a Youth who has brought a great deal of joy into my life. Crystal's birth to Mariah in January 1997 represented a challenging experience in its aftermath for her.

As I cherished my friendship with Crystal, I helped her as often as possible with Mariah. Babysitting her Daughter was a joy for me and my Parents. My Father was her "Playmate" on the living room floor. She would get on my Father's back, with his being in a four-point stance, and they would proceed to chant, " I am the King; I am the Queen!" My Mother's kindness was constantly shown in one way or another resulting in Mariah's seeing the value of others with respect to provided love. I was Mariah's surrogate "Aunt" who spent valuable time with her. Mariah's nickname for me was "Belby". Demonstrating that love and affection were not only relegated by Crystal, her Parent, but were willing opportunities that offered a personal giving from others in her young life, Mariah came to see that kindness came from the heart. Moreover, it was given freely and not from someone else's personal sacrifice. Mariah is a wonderful young Lady. She is intuitive, inquisitive, and places great value in the friendship of others. She will, one day, make a significantly important contribution to others because of her leadership and willingness to place the value of others above her own.

Our association has appeared to help Mariah to be a better individual. My disability has provided an appreciation in understanding the needs of others who suffer from debilitating physical deficiencies. Mariah sees my physical disability, but, at the same time, she does not acknowledge it. I am simply "Belby" to her and I am a friend who will always be there for her and she for me.

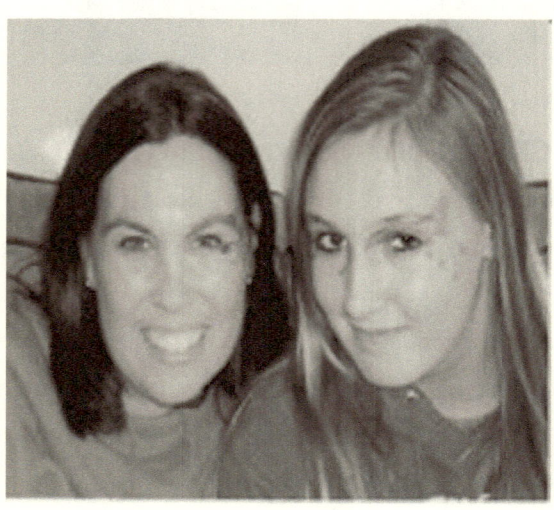

SHELLEY AND MARIAH

SHELLEY LYNN O'LEARY

JASON WEBSTER: My Cousin Jason was a huge factor in my life. He was often my Protector. Very often, there were situations when I was treated with little worth. Jason was always there for me, a Constant that offered a reminder that there were truly good people in the world, as he was and continues to be.

Jason "got" me. He understood me as to where I was coming from and he always accepted me for the disabled person that I was. In Junior High School, Jason would never hesitate to walk with me in the hallways. He always made me feel safe and entirely secure.

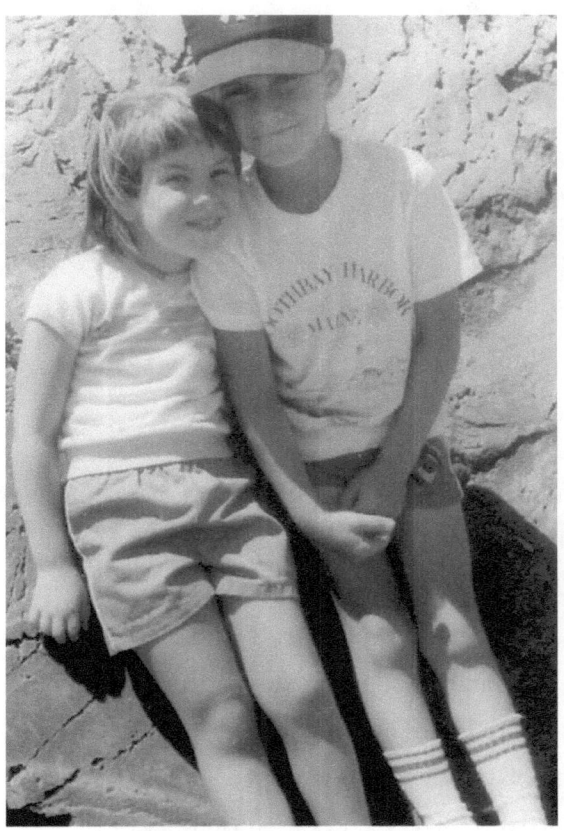

SHELLEY AND JASON

AMIE: Amie and I met some six or seven years ago. She has helped me through a lot with regard to my Dad's alcoholism. She always said that I did not give myself enough credit. I tell her that sometimes I feel "strange". She then replies that if I think it, then I am. As simplistic as that may sound, Amie is "right on". She is one of a few that I can count on for support in my life.

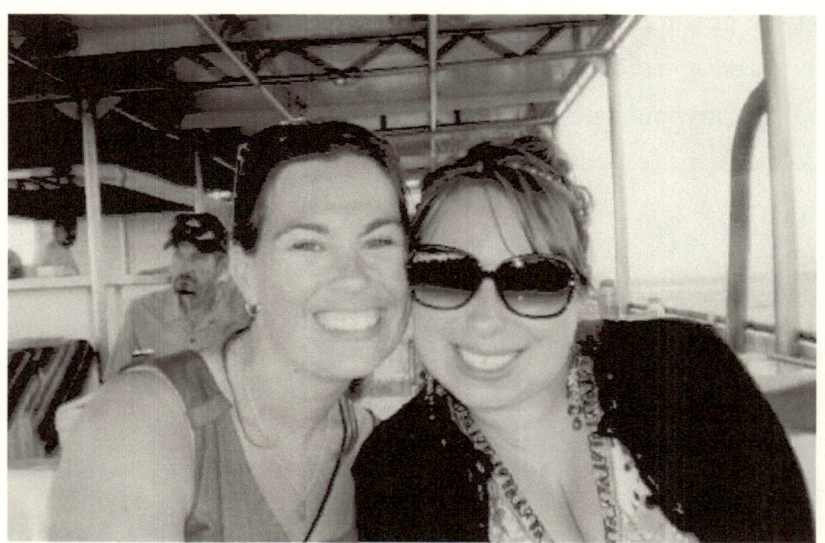

SHELLEY AND AMIE

MY GRANDFATHER "PAP": My Mother's Father was from Fort Kent, Maine and married my Grandmother who was brought up in New Brunswick, Canada. "Pap" served as a Navigator aboard B-24 Liberator Bomber Aircraft during World War II and flew 25 successful bombing missions from the English countryside before rotating back to the United States. He was a Graduate of Colby College and eventually became a very successful John Hancock Life Insurance Agent for many years. He was active in the Portland Civic Center as a Member of the Board of Directors and was a Member of the Masons.

SHELLEY LYNN O'LEARY

In 1989, he left our Town of Gorham when I was nine years old. He had had an affair with a woman from Long Island, New York and eventually divorced my Grandmother and married this other woman in September 1989 in the Boston area. He was never to live in Maine again prior to his death in 2010 in Saratoga Springs, New York. He and his wife made periodic trips to Gorham to visit my Parents over the years. Eventually, toward the end of his life, he was too frail to travel. His last visit to Maine was in 2009.

"Pap" was a kind and loving human being. He left his wife in Gorham at a time when he was needed the most in the up-bringing of my Cousin Jason who resided with my Grandparents at the time. It was a traumatic time for every member of the family and there are many who harbor less than positive feelings toward my Grandfather. However, we all know now and full-well that he is finally at peace.

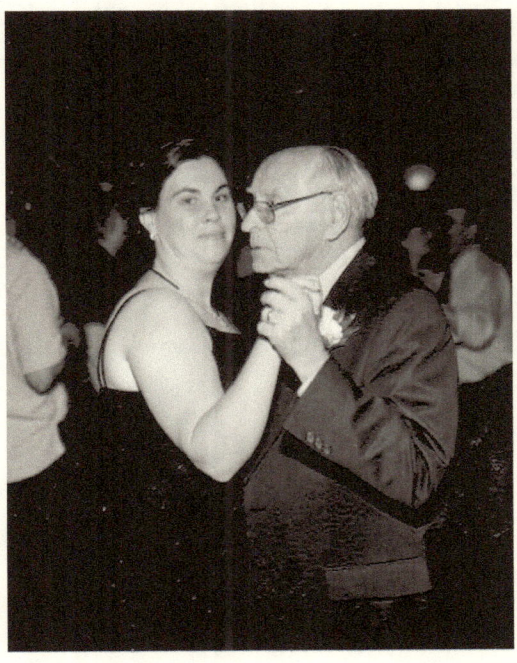

SHELLEY AND HER GRANDFATHER 'PAP'

MARY: Mary was the only true Friend I had in college. During my life, I "let in" very few individuals because of lack of trust in the knowledge that I would not be perceived as a "person of worth". It was difficult growing up with this feeling. Nevertheless, Mary was different. She understood me and more than empathized with my physical condition and my difficulty in learning. She was patient with my shortcomings. Whenever I needed her help, she was always there. In the final analysis of acknowledging friendships, Mary will always have a special place in my heart for her willingness to treat me as a person, and not one to be shunned, or pitied.

ANNIE: We met when I was working in Falmouth, Maine at Falmouth by the Sea, an assisted elderly home. This was during my internship when I was about to complete my Degree in Therapeutic Recreation from the University of Southern Maine in Portland in 2008. We have been Friends for two years. Annie has been instrumental in "bringing me out of my shell". As I have always been reluctant to engage with others socially, Annie showed me that my fear in doing so could be overcome with "taking a step slowly, one at a time" and chance to open up. As I did so, my confidence slowly built to the point that I am no longer the person who was somewhat intimidated to move forward in any friendly relationship. As with Crystal and Mary, Annie will always have a very special place in my heart for those who took their time to show me how to become a more complete person in every facet of my life.

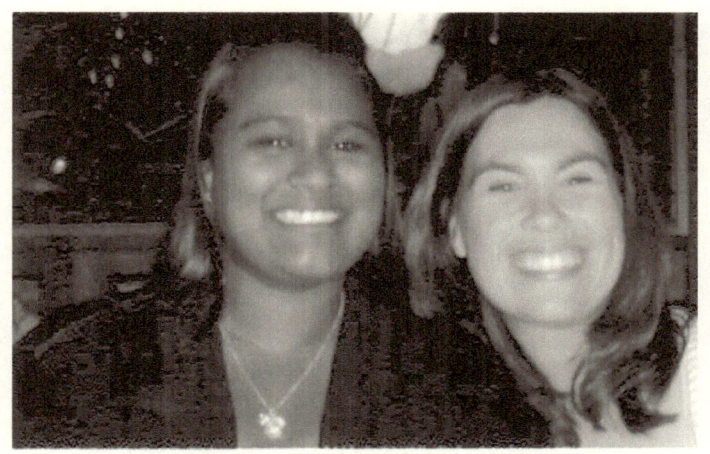

ANNIE AND SHELLEY

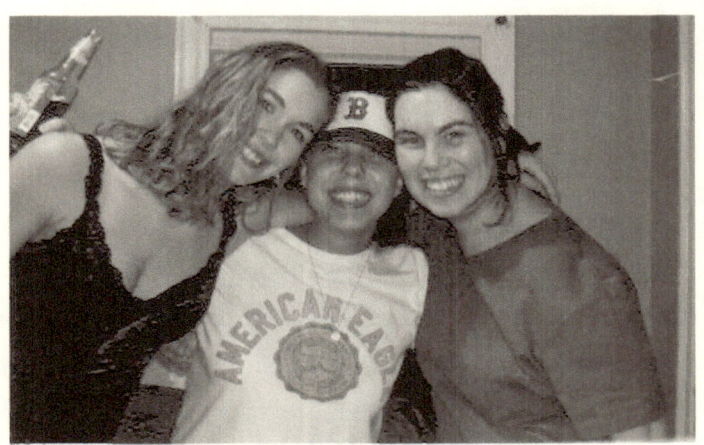

MARY AND KATRINA WITH SHELLEY

AUNT PEARL: My Aunt, my Grandfather's Sister, was somewhat of a model for me in that I saw her as the Family Protector of all this is right in the world. My Aunt didn't "take prisoners".

She told it like it was, with no embellishment, or desire to evade an issue. One knew where he or she stood with Aunt Pearl.

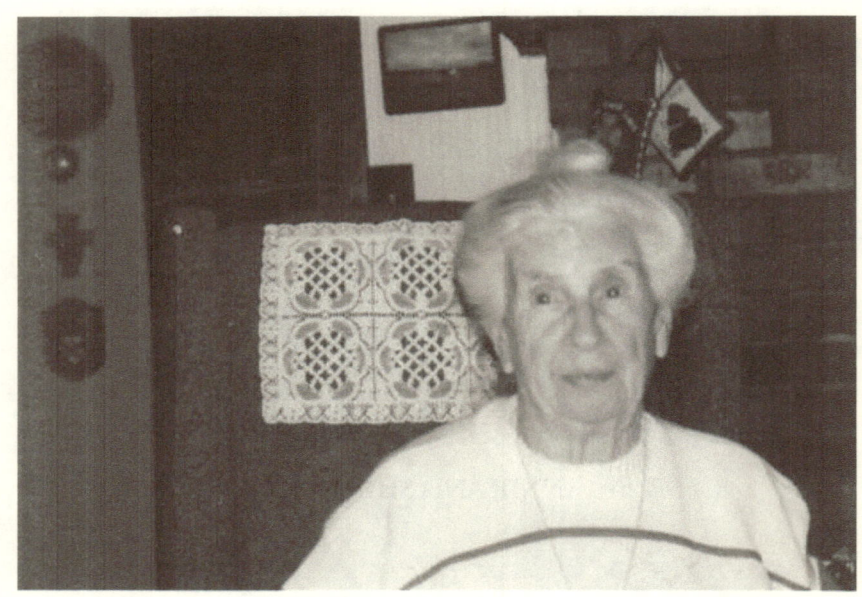

AUNT PEARL

She took her vows to become a Sister of Mercy and subsequently taught school at the first grade level. She was stern, but she was a fair "task master". She told you what was to be accomplished and her direction was crystal clear. She left no doubt as to her expectations. In addition, she was highly respected for her belief in treating everyone with more than an ounce of fairness. If you "screwed up", you understood why the resulting behavior modification was necessary. If you "shined", you took her praise as though it was a bag of gold because what she said or did was what was meant to be.

Aunt Pearl suffered an illness that resulted in the necessity to leave the Convent. I am told that she never lost that direction that she provided to many in her almost-90 years of life. She had that mischievous twinkle in her eye, much like her Father, my Great Grandfather Timothy James O'Leary, Sr.

SHELLEY LYNN O'LEARY

When her Mother Lillian passed away in the early 1970s, she took over the care and well-being of her Father. She did it willingly, and without reservation. There are those who may have said that the duty for Grampa's care should have fallen to Aunt Pearl as she was single, and no longer strictly affiliated with the Convent. My belief is that Aunt Pearl would have none of that conjecture and that she cared for her Father because she was devoted entirely to his care. She was the proverbial "Guardian Angel at the Gate", and fiercely protected my Great Grand-Father with every ounce of energy in her body.

When visiting with her every six months or so in Acushnet, Massachusetts, she would share with me her frustration in speaking to how she was enormously ignored by her sister's family, especially during the holiday season. It should be noted, in fairness to Aunt Fran, her Sister, that Aunt Pearl was consistently invited to participate in the Kennedy gatherings, and that she often declined such opportunity. For her reasons provided, it was never any one's place to judge. When my Great Grandfather was alive, the burden of travel falling on my Aunt Pearl's acceptance to travel to Cape Cod, the site of the familial gathering, was acknowledged in a gracious refusal. Grampa simply could not have withstood the rigors of travel by automobile as he was in his early 90's.

My relationship with Aunt Pearl could be considered as truly genuine. There appeared to be an "unspoken" understanding between us. She never judged me for my physical disability and always demonstrated patience with me as I would struggle to communicate my life's experiences. For that, I will always hold her in a very special place in my heart. Our meeting again after I leave this world will be one of true joy!

GREAT GRAMPA: My Dad's grandfather was a loving figure in my life. There are many pictures with me taken with him. I feel that in many ways we are kindred spirits and that oftentimes my decisions are based upon intuition that may only be explained by his spiritual presence. I believe that Aunt Pearl saw this for what it was, and, I would like to think that she was ultimately pleased with my apparent closeness to him. There were times when I would pass him by as he was resting his 90-year old body on the couch in the "sun room" at his Acushnet residence and I would stop before him, remove and pat his arm, and walk off. These tender moments, however fleeting, were an indication of a love that we had for one another. Great Grampa was a World War I Hero who fought in France with the Famous Fighting 69th Irish Division. He was yards away when the famous Poet Joyce Kilmer was killed. Great Grampa was reputed to wear the smallest uniform in the Army at the time.

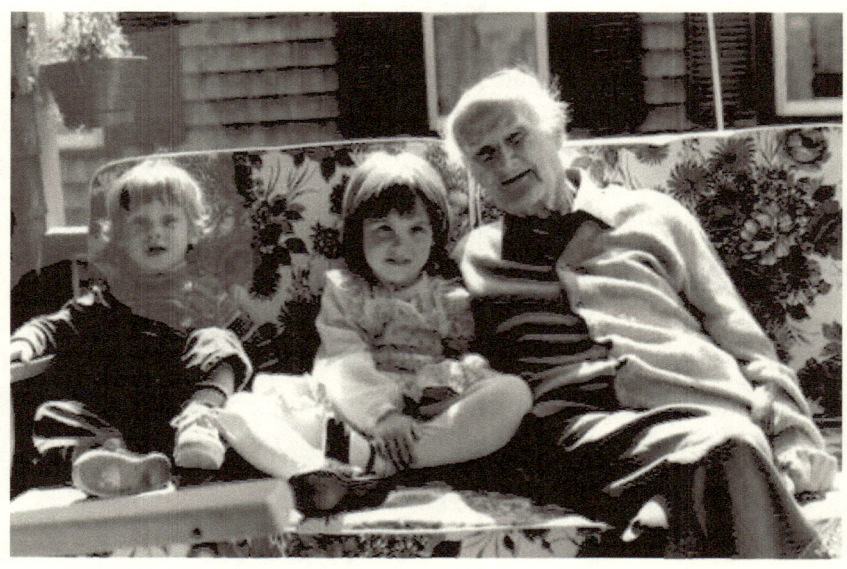

GREAT GRAMPA WITH TIMMY AND SHELLEY

My disability defines who I am. It speaks to my acknowledgement of a fear that I may never be able to measure up in meeting new challenges that are afforded to others without my disability.

And it's a type of fear that makes me feel that I am all alone in my understanding of who I am, representing a strong emotion that comes over me when I least expect it. I have always had the feeling that no one "gets me" or understands what I go through every day of my life. It is a life's "haunting" that never stops.

My disability affects my relationships with others in that I am somewhat of an "ugly duckling" in a pond of "beauty" that I can never match. This anxiety of solitude lends itself to the emotion that others will never accept me for the inner beauty that I am without my shadow of disability always behind me, always chasing me, almost mocking me, and never letting me be viewed as a "normal". Will I always be alone?

I dream sometime of walking on a beach with someone who loves me for whom I am. I envision this person holding my left hand and not having the feeling of revulsion at "comforting" my disability with unconditional love in his heart. It would be as if he is not holding me per se, but he is cradling my disability and loving it for what it is. That to me is a definition of a "soul mate". That to me is loving my being and accepting me without reservation and without prejudice for an outward projection of my inner true self.

CUDDLES: One of life's most significant blessings is the company of a pet. Cuddles was a tiger cat that we picked up from an Animal Refuge League shelter in August 1986. She was so scrawny that I fell in love with her immediately. Cuddles was eight weeks old when we brought her home and she enriched our lives for the next 17 years.

This cat was a favorite to us all, although my Father would never admit to that fact. She would have her way of working her way into one's heart that was altogether endearing. Dad professed his disdain for cats and would

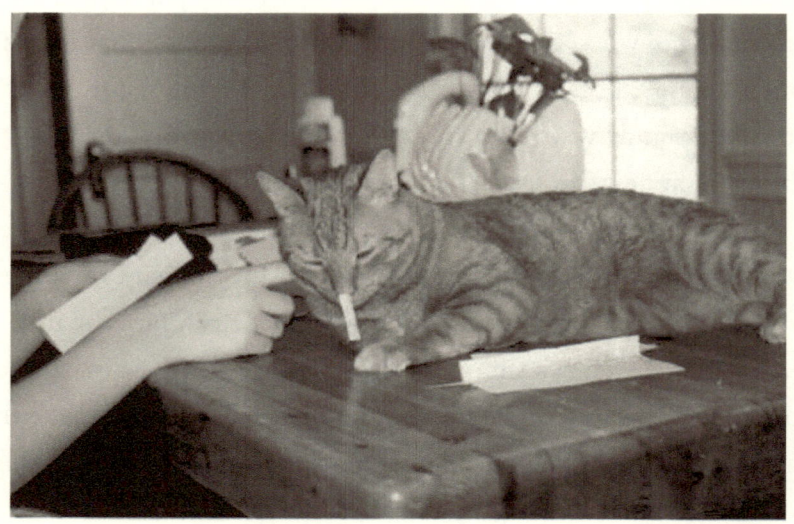

CUDDLES IN A FRISKY MOMENT

have nothing to do with her at first while declaring that Cuddles was mine and mine alone. Cats are funny in one respect. They sense a human's dislike, and tend to polarize immediately to that one person who cannot stand to have a cat being around him. Cuddles, of course, was no exception with my Father as he was sitting on the couch. Cuddles would immediately jump into his lap and commence with the loudest "purring" and/or "snoring". Dad would never be mean to any animal and he soon took to petting Cuddles on a consistent basis while she would settle herself comfortably on his lap.

Over the years, it appeared that Cuddles would be jealous of Mom and Dad sitting beside one another on the couch as they watched television.

SHELLEY LYNN O'LEARY

Cuddles would jump up onto the couch, look my Mom in the eye, and "worm" her way between my parents and settle against my Father. She would then begin to "purr" while looking up at my Mother as if to suggest that "he was all mine"! Needless to say, this was the entertainment for the evening.

Cuddles was a definite feline of habit! Each night, she would wait for all of us to go to bed. Cuddles would sit in the hall at about the same time each evening and wait for Mom and Dad to get into bed. She would make sure that they were comfortably settled in before coming into my room. She would then jump onto my bed and settle herself on my pillow, satisfied in the "knowledge" that all was well with the O'Leary's for that night.

When Cuddles reached her 17th year, she developed tumors that affected her concentration. My Dad would find her in the middle of the upstairs hallway and simply stare vacantly ahead. When we took her to the Vet, he checked her tumors and suggested that it was time to put her out of her misery. This was very difficult for me, and I saw very hard for my Father as well.

On the day that Cuddles was taken to the Vet, my Dad volunteered to go with me. After the shots administered to her, the Vet kindly remarked that she was no longer suffering. I know I shed many tears that day and I know that Dad also felt terribly sad as well.

We took her ashes a few days later and buried them beside a fence in our backyard. We had a bronze plaque made up that had her name and the years of her life inscribed. All of us will never forget the tremendous joy this wonderful animal brought to all of us. And after she left us, I would "feel" her presence, especially when I was going through a sad period. This would serve to comfort me in my time of need.

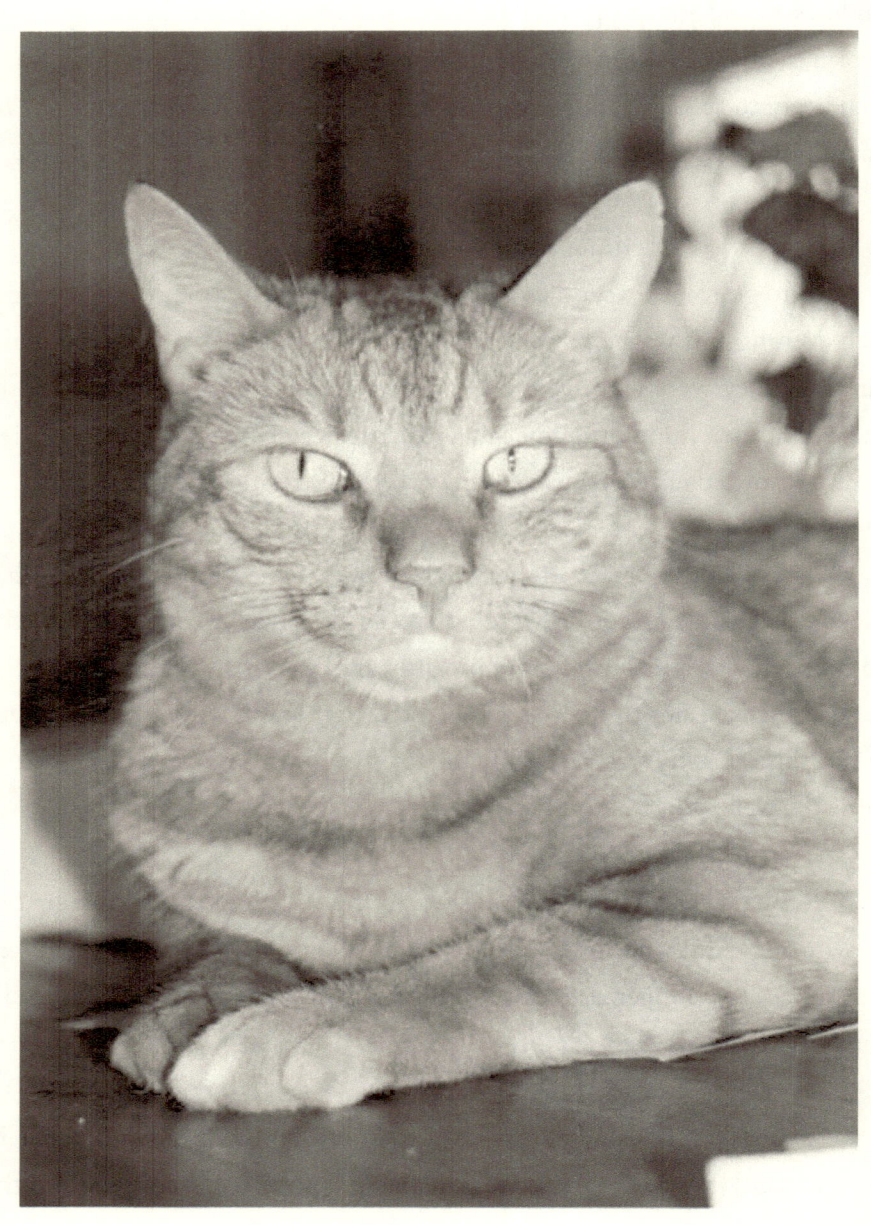

CUDDLES

SEIZURES AND PANIC ATTACKS

I WAS TOLD THAT my Parents suspected my first seizures visibly occurring when we were visiting with my Grandfather and Aunt Pearl in Acushnet, Massachusetts. I was two years old. My Father walked into their living room to find out what I was doing and he saw me lying on my back on the carpet. I was very still and staring vacantly up at the ceiling. My Dad called to me to ask if I was all right, and I did not respond at first. Then, I "snapped" out of it and turned toward him. He said later that I reacted to him as if nothing had happened.

From that moment on, I continued to have "small" episodic seizures, or "*petit mal*" occurrences. It was not until I was eight or nine when I experienced my first "*grand mal*" seizure, as defined by the experienced mentioned at the outset of my book. Of course, this is not to say with one-hundred assurances that I did not go through previous major physical ones without my realizing it, or for anyone else seeing them to occur. The possibility was always there. Seizures came with the "territory" due to my brain injury suffered at birth.

Having a seizure is *not* fun! An individual, who experiences one, is paralyzed and cannot do anything about it. It begins with a "funny" feeling, sometimes accompanied by a "tingling" sensation. Oftentimes, there is a feeling that an "elephant" is sitting on your chest! You cannot move. Simply speaking, you cannot do anything about what is going to happen next.

The uncontrollable body spasms come next. When I have them, I cannot communicate. My hearing and sight are alive and take everything in around me. I see those who attempt to comfort me, and I hear the frustration and anxiety in the voices of those who want to do something to help me. It is scary for individuals witnessing an episode because there is a feeling of complete helplessness. People, who are not accustomed to seeing someone go through a seizure, try to be proactive and attempt "remedial" measures that simply do not apply in these situations. There is a lack of understanding in the "mechanics" of immediate care.

My parents went through this phase in their misunderstanding of "helping" me to overcome my experience. In time, and with wise counsel by someone like Dr. Walter Allan, the appropriate action to take is to keep the person from injuring himself. If, after a certain amount of time has elapsed with the affected person still "seizing", then specific action to seek care by calling in health-care professionals may be necessary.

When the seizure has run its course, it leaves the person feeling tremendously fatigued! Being "washed out" is a term that is entirely applicable. There is emptiness in terms of energy level. All one wants to do is sleep. It is amazing what a *"grand mal"* seizure can do to a person's desire to be active, or the desire to lie down and "sleep for a week"!

As experiencing a seizure is quite unlike a favorite cone of ice cream, a person who has had enough of them knows that impending seizures create what are known as "panic attacks" in their anticipation. These attacks occur when a "notion" arises that reminds the epileptic that such a "feeling" is a one-hundred percent precursor that a seizure is imminent.

SHELLEY LYNN O'LEARY

This "feeling" is not, however, in reality, a guarantee that a person will actually have a seizure. If the resulting moments following a panic attack do not result in any epileptic episode, it does not necessarily mean that the person can easily dismiss the prior anticipated intuition that he has "dodged the bullet". On the contrary, it promotes a sense of "doom" being right around the corner.

Each time a panic attack occurs, it leaves a small "emotional scar" in one's psyche. This panic attack experience, or "scar", is then provoked repeatedly when a certain set of circumstance occur to serve as a "trigger" for the panic attack. It is an on-going cycle. The more fearful the seizure, the higher the level of apprehension for having another or subsequent one. This, then, translates into a corresponding measure of intensity regarding panic attacks.

Any daily experience that may relate back to panic, in one form or another, systematically creates or sets off a "trigger" for that panic. It also "opens a window" for the onset of a seizure either big or small. It is important for one to know how "to close that window" so that the specter of a seizure cannot work its way into one's emotional well-being.

I have since learned "to trick" my brain by leaving the lights and/or radio on at night. These actions appear "to satisfy" my brain into "believing" that all is well with the world and that it is "time" to let go of all anxiety at that moment in time.

My Mother found a woman neurologist who was conducting research regarding the possibility of isolating the portion of the brain that caused seizures. After an extensive meeting with the neurologist, my parents decided that it was well worth the effort to determine if her theories about brain damage and the resulting seizures were valid. It was decided that I would spend several days at the Maine Medical Center for the testing.

The idea was for me to ignore purposely the taking of my seizure-resistant medications to induce a *grand-mal* event. This, of course, was a major concern for me as I had gone through these type of seizures in the past. I was not looking forward to the prospect of going through another one!

My Father spent a couple of nights in my hospital room and slept on a cot. When I eventually experienced the seizure, my Dad tried to get the nurse on-station to come to the room and take care of my situation. It took several moments for a nurse to arrive. My Father was not too happy about the lack of immediate medical response.

During the seizure, my brain-wave patterns were monitored and documented on tape. In the final analysis, there was not enough data collected to ascertain the proper remedial response to the seizure. It was an exercise with no solution.

Even though nothing, in essence, came from my stay in the hospital, the need to pursue this alternative toward correcting my physical deficiency was a step that needed to be taken. There was the hope that the seizure that was self-induced would shed some light on where exactly the electrical brain impulses occurred so that this portion of the brain could be identified for subsequent testing and possible repair. It was not to be, however.

SHELLEY LYNN O'LEARY

POWERFUL AND TEACHABLE MOMENTS

MY PERSONAL ATTACK: When I was 18 years old, I was assaulted by someone I trusted. The experience shook me to the core. I honestly feel that I will never fully recover from the emotional impact, although I have learned to live with the knowledge that it did happen. It has been important for me to address the occurrence psychologically and emotionally. For me to ignore that it took place would result in stifling a memory that would one-day return to harm me emotionally. It is akin to a sleeping tiger cub. To ignore this animal for several years is to ignore the danger that this tiger, now fully grown, represents relative to a much more significant threat to my well-being. Whereas a tiger cub may snap, a fully-grown tiger may devour. I felt for a very long time that I would never be able to will myself "to get over" what had happened to me. The fact that I am able to address what happened is a positive step in my emotional and psychological recovery. Having empowered myself to choose to live my life in a meaningful way in the aftermath permits me to accept the occurrence for what it was. In addition, in that light, I feel a sense of peace through my ability to let it go. Even though I feel at peace, I still struggle with trusting men.

I have not been able to accomplish my present and tranquil mental and emotional state of mind without the help of my good Friend, Lois. She has been invaluable as a resource in assisting me to overcome a sense of despair.

Lois' wisdom and guidance have provided me with the appropriate and necessary direction to take charge of my life and not let the negative aspects of what life offers rule over my desire to seek what happiness that life may offer. Both Lois and my doctor have been instrumental in assuring me that I was not a victim, but merely an "instrument of circumstance".

MY AUTOMOBILE ACCIDENTS: Some additional powerful moments that will remain with me for the rest of my life were two accidents involving automobiles. One was when I was riding my bicycle as a seven-year old. The other was when I was a driver of my Honda CRV Sport Utility Vehicle.

After learning how to ride my bike, I was allowed to take it to school one day. My elementary school was located across our busy State Highway in front of our house and some 300 yards farther down the road. After school, I arrived at the crossover point in front of our home. I was forbidden to ride my bicycle across the street due to the very high volume of daily traffic. I was told to look both ways and walk the bike across the street to the top of our driveway. As the way was clear in both directions, I proceeded to cross the road. At the same time, my mother was in her Honda Accord and was in the process of backing out of our driveway. I hurried across the road and fell in the "blind spot" of my Mother's view as she was backing up.

All of a sudden, I was struck by the rear of Mom's car and thrown to the ground. My Mother continued backing up and all of a sudden stopped abruptly. At this point, she had no idea that she had hit me and that I was lying under the rear bumper and against her rear tires. The manifold exhaust from the Honda was pressing down on my chest, and I was pinned and could not move.

SHELLEY LYNN O'LEARY

My little Brother Timmy was strapped into the back seat. When my Mother stopped the car she thought she heard a metal scraping sound, as if she had run over some metal device. She immediately turned back to Timmy and asked anxiously, "Where's Shelley?" Timmy responded that he had no idea where she was.

My Mother immediately got out of the car and found me pinned under the car. I then asked her, "Mom, why did you run hit/over me?" My Mother panicked. She had almost run over her Daughter and killed her. The bicycle was across the street, and on the sidewalk.

The strange thing about the occurrence was: why did my Mother stop backing up? She swore that she and Timmy heard her vehicle hit something behind her, but it could not have been the bike because of its location on the opposite side of the street and on the sidewalk. There was no other metal device anywhere near the rear of the vehicle. Only Shelley was there and pinned under the car! The only thing that they could come up with was that a miracle had occurred that spared my life. My Mother was somehow warned not to continue to move the car in reverse because I was in her blind spot right behind the Honda and she never saw me. She hit me and I went down. Somehow, that day was not the day for me to leave this earth!

On another occasion, I was driving my Honda CRV from Gorham and into Portland to meet my Dad at the Department of Human Services. I was not use to the side streets in Portland, but decided to take one of them as a shortcut to the Human Services location. There were two stop signs, one right after the other, for me to stop on one of the side streets. I saw the first one and completely ran through the second. I got to the middle of that intersection and I was broadsided by a vehicle that had the right of way. Fortunately, I and the other driver was not injured, but I was pretty shaken up. I could have died that day, but I truly believe God had other plans for me in the future.

Of course, my automobile experiences were not solely relegated to very serious consequences. Soon after I graduated from Gorham High School, my Parents surprised me by buying me a new Saturn for a graduation gift. They took me over to the dealership and I was presented with a red Saturn that had a huge bow on the hood. I was excited.

After the paperwork was signed, I drove my new car back to our house. I pulled into the driveway and before bringing the car to a stop, I sideswiped a tree that stood near the side of the driveway. Contact with the tree cause my driver's side-view mirror to break off! I was mortified! My Father saw what I had done, smiled, shook his head, and went into the house. He came out a few moments later with a roll of duct tape and proceeded to affix the detached mirror to the car. I could only be me!

On another occasion not too very long after I got my driver's license, I was out driving with a couple of friends. On the way home, I let one of them, who did not have her license, drive my car back to Gorham. Well, her father was a police officer with the Gorham Police Department. Somehow, he found out about her daughter's unauthorized driving and came over to our home. He mentioned what had happened to my Parents and he left it for them to deal with the issue.

My Father proceeded to take my license away for six months. At the end of six months, I did not come forward to ask to have it back. In fact, it was a whole year before I approached my Father about getting my license back. He told me that he was wondering when I would be asking him for it because the suspension was good for only a half-year!

SHELLEY LYNN O'LEARY

MY WORK EXPERIENCE

FALMOUTH BY THE SEA: Prior to my graduation with my Associate's Degree in Therapeutic Recreation, I was assigned by the University of Southern Maine and my Advisor to do an internship at an assisted elderly home in Falmouth, Maine. It is truly then when my adult "work" experience began. Although there were trials experienced during this relatively brief period, I learned a lot about myself in helping the elderly to ease through their daytime living. I was expected to take the initiative in many situations after a "feeling out" period by my supervisory staff member. Eventually, the comfort level settled in and I felt more at ease. I looked forward to seeing a few of the elderly on a daily basis.

One woman in particularly was "E". She was a gentle soul who always went out of her way to acknowledge my presence, despite her Parkinson's disability. Of all of the elderly, "E" was probably the woman that I missed the most after I left Falmouth by the Sea.

I also gave my extra time freely to assist in any way I could to lighten the load of my supervisor's periodic scheduling dilemma, whom I knew to be appreciative of my willingness to help.

During this time, I assisted in supervising bingo activities, which I have to admit were "lively" and highly competitive. I secretly developed a motto that suggested I should never stand in the way or block an elderly woman's bingo card! I valued my life too much!

I was also tasked with leading a Prayer service on Sundays. In addition, there were opportunities to take the elderly on brief out-of-home excursions that were entirely enjoyable. My supervisor was just incredible in helping me to make the initial adjustment to the work environment, as well as allowing me to use my good judgment in supervising activities. Overall, I learned a lot from this internship and I truly feel that it assisted in molding me to be the person who saw the need in others and to do something about that need.

THE MORRISON CENTER: Employment opportunities were truly at a premium when I finally got my Associates' Degree in Therapeutic Recreation from the University of Southern Maine. I considered myself extremely fortunate to be accepted for the position at the Center that assisted in providing educational, emotional, and supervisory direction to many children who came to Morrison with varying levels of needy attention.

One five-year old captured my "heart". I refer to him in this recounting as "S". His condition was such that he had difficulty "trusting" anyone who served to intrude upon his "well-being". In time and with more than an ounce of love and caring, "S" began to open up to me to the extent that no other staff member was able to achieve like results. Working with "S" on a daily basis and seeing his responsiveness to my attempts to touch his inner concerns with love and true caring were personal joys. Yes, these were occupational accomplishments and break-throughs. They represented only a beginning for "S" living in his "inside world", coupled with his willingness to experience an "outside relationship" with those around him. My Mother was amazed at how well I was able to relate to "S", a child struggling with autism. She has referred to me as the "Child Whisperer"!

Of course, Morrison employment also presented itself with many, diverse, and unique challenges. Not only was it difficult to deal with behavioral considerations, but there was always a fear I had that I would have to re-live my own seizure experience by watching a child go through his own. I was fortunate by the time of this recounting that I witnessed only two occasions where a child or fellow colleague suffered through one of those episodes.

At the Morrison Center, a special kind of person had to be present on a daily basis, one who was resilient to accept behavioral changes in the children who loved you one moment and were overtly and physically challenging the next. It was not unusual for a child with behavioral concerns to lash out at me or another counselor. The task was to find the point in that child's discontent, in that snapshot in time, and to deal with it spontaneously and effectively in a way that the child "learned" from the outburst. This "corrective" treatment measure was always meant to show understanding and to impart an avenue of awareness of what the child had done. In addition, it offered a solution to the existing problem that the child could deal with and accept, thereby diminishing an escalation to "out of control". It was during these "behavior modification" exercises that the thought would come to mind that the "weekend couldn't come soon enough"!

There were many opportunities to "laugh" at myself in the performance of my duties. I was not known for my balance, for example, especially when getting on a swing in the playground area. When trying to get going, I would invariably fall off! I would just shrug and tell myself "I had to be me!" There was another time in Arts & Crafts when I got watercolor paint all over me! Trying to downplay that this was my true "artistic self" surfacing was not enough for everyone else to believe me, or to stop giggling at my artistic expression!

The Falmouth-by-the-Sea and the Morrison Center experiences have helped me to be a better person. At both venues, I have been praised for my ability to reach out and help someone else with his immediate problem. This is truthfully no great mystery for me. There is something down deep in my soul that begs me to extend my devotion toward helping others who need physical and emotion direction in their lives. As I continue to enjoy my relationship with these children, I see myself growing, not so much as an employee, but more so as an individual who is able to make a difference in another child's life. If I can reach out and touch another individual in need and have that person become one who sees himself as a better person of worth, then I have achieved a worthwhile and significant accomplishment.

There have been moments in my life when I have been able to impart my message of hope to others who have suffered as I have, or more intensely.

THE EPILEPSY FOUNDATION: I was provided an opportunity to share my experience as an Epileptic with a colleague of mine during an interview by a television news channel host. My colleague and I have been Members of a Foundation that works tirelessly to bring to the attention of the Maine people that Epilepsy is an emotionally painful experience and requires the awareness of everyone. Our first State Dinner held in Portland, Maine in November 2011 served as a springboard to communicate with the public at large that Epilepsy is a condition that is alive and well. Further

SHELLEY LYNN O'LEARY

research is required to help discover new medicinal treatment opportunities for those who suffer from this debilitating condition.

The Maine Foundation has also sponsored Walks to advertise that Epilepsy is to be recognized and that it is not going away. On the contrary, these group exercises have served to announce that continuous monetary support is required to further Epilepsy awareness. In addition, all of the Foundation activities are representations in terms of imparting to the people of Maine that important research is on-going to achieve ultimate results to be shared by those afflicted. The time for results cannot arrive soon enough!

MY RELATIONSHIPS WITH FAMILY AND FRIENDS

WHEN MY BROTHER Michael would bring some of his friends over to the house, I usually made it a point to interrupt anything that they were doing. He had some of the "cutest" guys come over to the house. Of course, my interruptions were not lost on my Brother. He always knew exactly what I was doing!

One of the great things about Holidays was the time spent with family together. Thanksgiving was always a fun time. After our holiday meal, those of us who could "push ourselves away from the table", would go outside and play a game of touch football. At first, the playing involved my two Brothers, my Cousin Jason, and my Father. In later years, my Brother Michael's three children would join the fun and give everyone a "run for his money". My two Nephews and my Niece would run the "old people" ragged.

There was one Thanksgiving when we had an early snowfall of four inches two days prior to the Holiday. The ensuing two days were just beautiful, though, and six of us went out and played in the "Snow Bowl" in our backyard after eating. On one play, my feet went out from under me and I went down. I slid about six feet before coming to a stop! It was not the "play of the day", but it provided great comic relief!

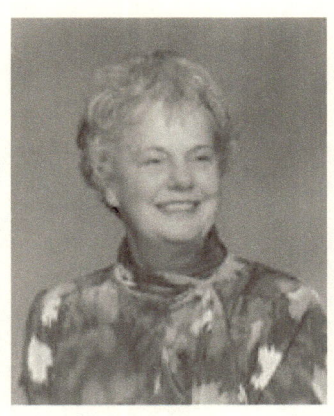

MY MATERNAL GRANDMOTHER

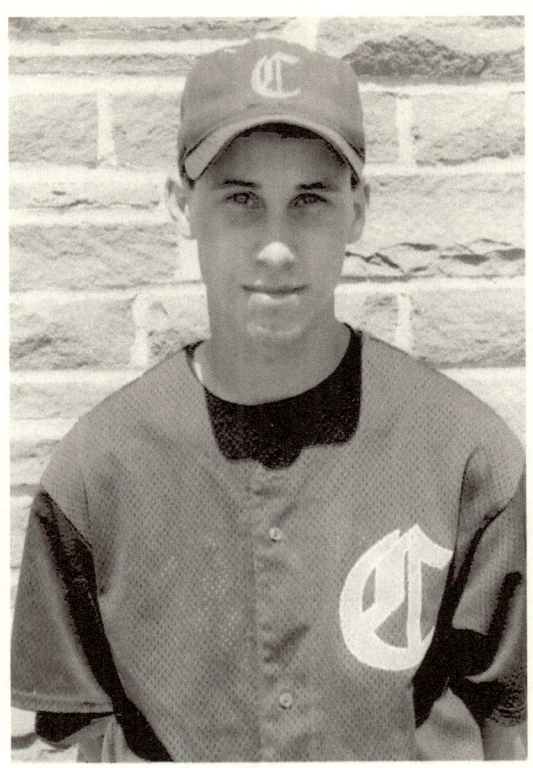

MY BROTHER TIMMY, A CLEMSON GRADUATE

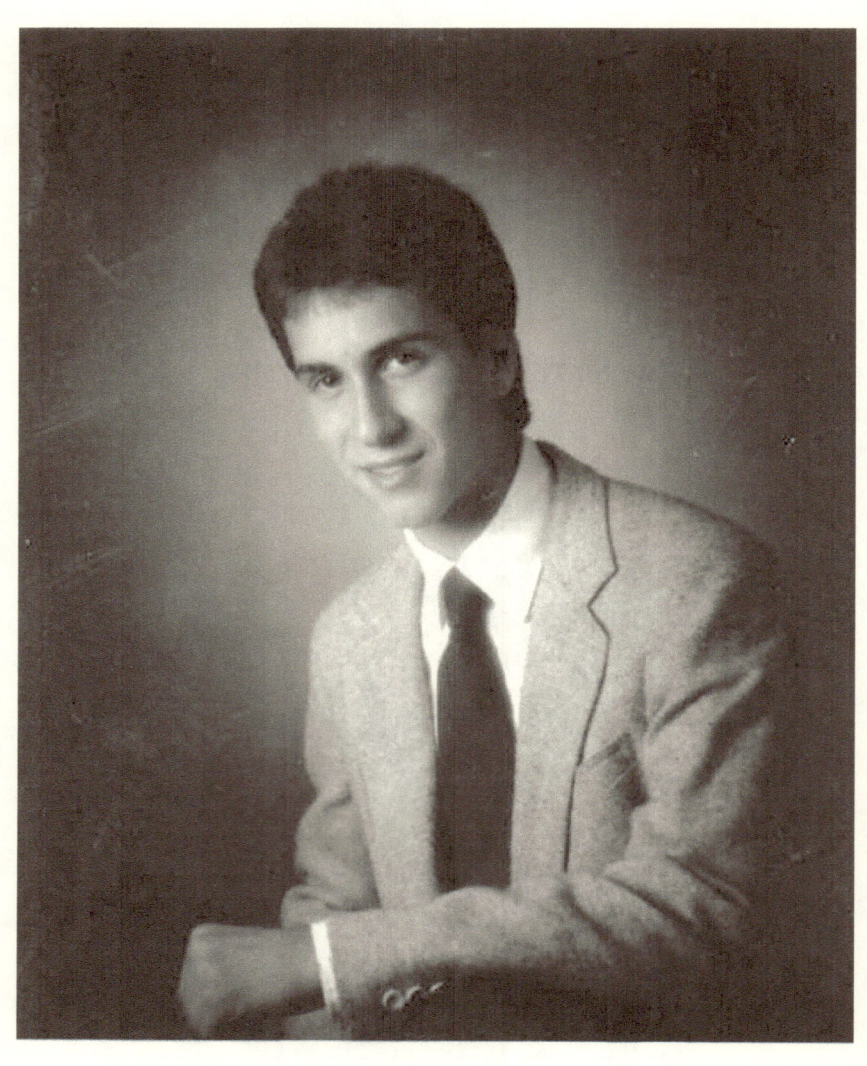

MY BROTHER MICHAEL, BOSTON COLLEGE GRADUATE

Christmas morning was a wonderful time for all of us. Quite often, it was a time of waiting when I was older and my younger Brother Timmy was still living in the house. He would love to sleep late and we would let him so that our anticipation could continue to build regarding the giving of gifts.

Our holiday meals were usually shared with my Grandmother and my Aunt who lived a half-mile from our home. My Grandmother had this wonderfully-tasting Jell-O-like concoction, green in color and filled with different fruit. To date, I am hoping that I may be able talk her out of her recipe. My older Brother Michael, who lived in nearby Yarmouth, would come over the day after the official holiday with my Nephews and Niece. In the last couple of years, we would see very little of my younger Brother Timmy who had moved to Charleston, South Carolina.

Both of my Brothers have always been supportive of me in anything I would do or attempt to do. They have been receptive to whenever I found the time to talk to them about what was going on in my life. I know that my life has been somewhat of a struggle; but, I also know that if I ever needed my Brothers to help me, they would never hesitate to be there for me.

I have briefly mentioned my Friend Amie early in this Book. She has really been someone who has truly listened to my concerns. This has come into play when I would speak about my Father's alcoholism. She always had the appropriate words to share. Her confidence put me at ease for the most part. Amie's fellowship has always been supportive. We also had the occasion to travel to Cabo San Lucas together for a week to celebrate her graduation from college. This was a most enjoyable trip.

Crystal has also been mentioned earlier. She and I have had many fun times together. Whether they were on a cruise or in the mountains skiing, we have always enjoyed one another's company. Being associated with her Daughter Mariah has been a blessing for me.

I have dated rarely. There was one individual whom I saw for a couple of years. I will refer to him as "J". We went to movies and simply hung out together. Our relationship could not really be labeled as "serious", although I truly liked "J" a lot. He was several years younger than I was. His commitment to a long-term serious relationship just was not there because I felt that he was not ready to jump into one. My Mother always told me that my time would come with spending the rest of my life with a married partner. Everything works out for a reason.

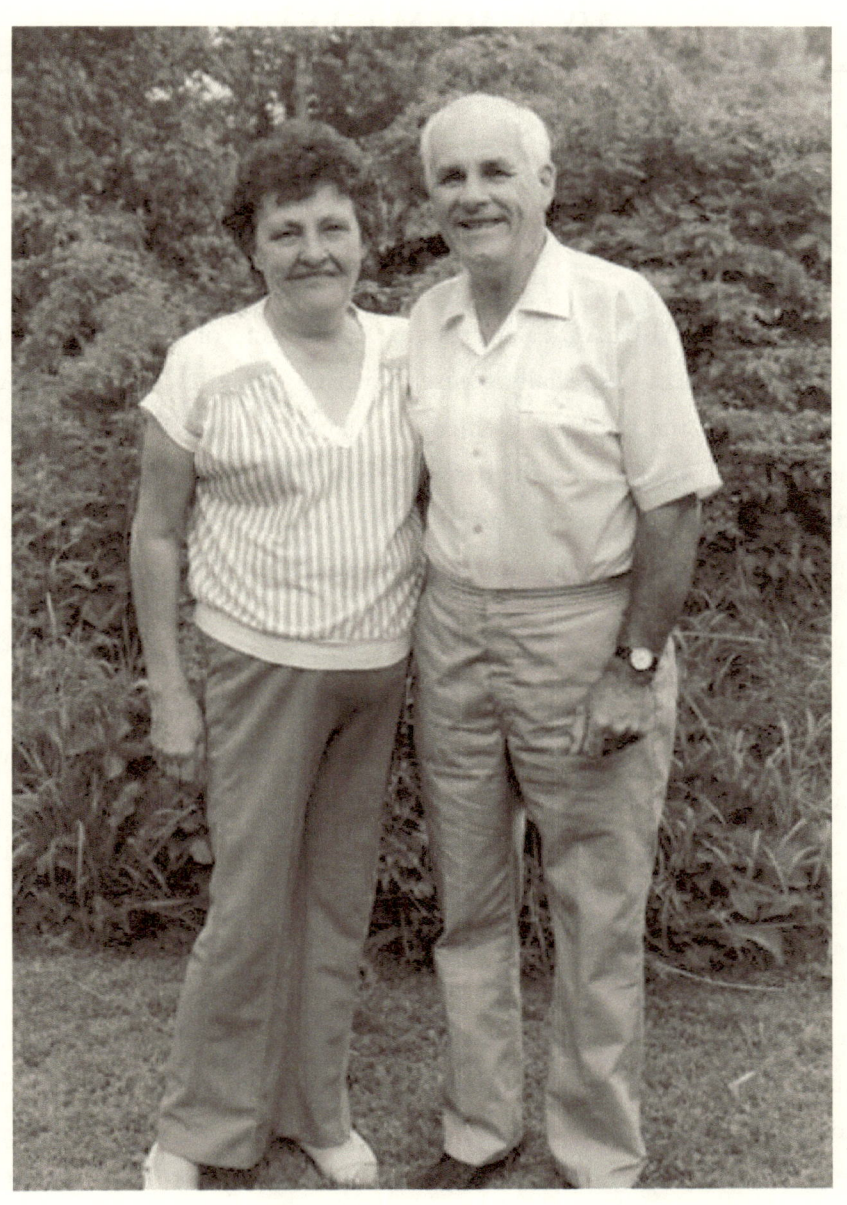

MY PATERNAL GRANDPARENTS

MY ACADEMIC YEARS

I HAVE ALREADY addressed a portion of my educational experiences, especially those affecting Title IX responsibilities imposed upon the Gorham Elementary School System. During my high school years, I was put into the Resource Room for students who displayed difficulty in learning. I have to admit that I could have fought to stay out of that category because I really did have the ability to grasp various concepts in all of my classes.

One particular episode comes to mind when I was asked by my Resource Room teacher if I knew what an exclamation point was. I was incensed that I had to be asked such a question. Of course, I knew what an exclamation point was! I was so peeved that I asked myself, "How dare they ask me that question!"

This was but the tip of the iceberg, however. There were many others what I considered "insulting" moments during my high school years. It created in me a lack of self-confidence. When one gets to that point, it often leads to a feeling that maybe other perceptions of me are accurate. Maybe I really do have a learning disability. It was not until years of being told by my Mother that I really did have the ability to learn when I began to see myself in a different cognitive light. In addition, her insistence that I could succeed in the classroom led me to want to pursue a college education.

I was admitted to Andover College in Portland a few years after my high school graduation. I had this intense desire to prove that I was worthy of acquiring a college degree. Both my Brothers had their Bachelor's Degrees in Economics, Mike at Boston College in 1991, and Timmy at Clemson University in 2005. There was not any reason why I could not achieve the same milestone.

Therefore, I set my sights on getting an Associate's Degree in Business Administration at Andover. My study habits were virtually non-existent, but my Mother once again helped me to learn in my own way. Her patience was outstanding. When I had to go into the hospital for a week of tests relating to my epilepsy, my Father got permission from my professor to sit in on a couple of classes for me so that I wouldn't fall too far behind. He sat down with me and went over the Microsoft Excel information after I was released from Maine Medical. I felt that I had not skipped a beat.

My graduation was one of the happiest days of my life. We celebrated at our home and many of my friends came over to share in my accomplishment, to include Susan-Cody Butler. It was more than generous for her to share her time with me and to acknowledge my accomplishment.

After my graduation, I worked as a Swim Instructor at the Rieche Pool. Karen, my Supervisor, talked to me about going for my degree in therapeutic recreation. She told me that my future work would always be in working with the physically-challenged and that getting my degree would make me more marketable in the job market. It made perfect sense to me.

Therefore, I talked to my parents and they agreed to help me to get through the program conducted at the University of Southern Maine. I was able to get credit for some of my work from my Business Administration Associate's Degree Program and so I had 12 courses to take before I could qualify for my Associate's in Therapeutic Recreation. I took one to two courses at a time and at the end of two and a half years, I graduated with my second Associate's Degree. I'll always thank Karen for getting me on the right track, as well as my Mother who helped me every step of the way. This second graduation celebration was one that I will always savor. The entire experience taught me that I could achieve my educational goals despite the difficult learning hurdles I had to overcome.

SHELLEY LYNN O'LEARY

MY ATHLETIC ACTIVITIES

I HAVE ALWAYS ENJOYED swimming. This was an activity that I could manage quite well despite my disability affecting my left side. I started taking lessons when I was five years old and had wonderful Instructors. Karen was one who was always understanding and patient with me. My experience led me to eventually teach others with physical challenges in the pool at the Rieche School in Portland. I was very self-competitive. I always told myself that there wasn't anything I couldn't accomplish in the water because I was always insistent on succeeding regardless how difficult the task was in front of me!

My ability to swim with a near-perfect stroke, limited only by my left-side partial paralysis, was noticed by my employers. They eventually asked me to demonstrate this stroke to others who were physically-challenged in the water. As swimming gave me an edge in doing things that others without physical disabilities would not do, I pursued this exercise by competing for my Senior Life Saving Badge. I acquired it as a teenager. My experience swimming taught me responsibility and respect for water. To this day, I am ever mindful of the dangers that the ocean, lake, or a swimming pool present to others who take being in the water for granted.

When I was five years old, my Mother signed me up to take gymnastic lessons. This proved to be excellent physical therapy for me as it assisted in my maintaining appropriate balance during the course of normal living.

These lessons lasted about one year. Even today, my Instructor, Mr. Marston, remembers me as the little girl who refused to give up and accepted any and all challenges, especially with negotiating the balance beam.

My Mother, ever the one to seize the opportunity to help me through my physical disability soon had me involved with dance classes. These were a lot of fun for me. I had the opportunity to wear my own dance "uniform" and perform a recital with several others in my class. Once again, this activity lasted about a year.

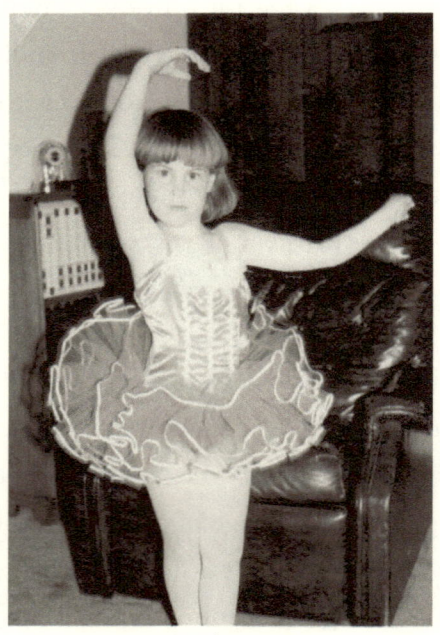

SHELLEY'S DANCE CLASS

I took up skiing when I became acquainted with the Maine Handicap Skiing Program. My Mother and I would go up to the Sunday River Ski Resort and spend the day skiing the slopes with other physically-challenged children. Once again, my Instructors were simply fabulous. This lasted two years. Later, I had an occasion to go skiing with Crystal and her family who enjoyed navigating the slopes often during the winter months.

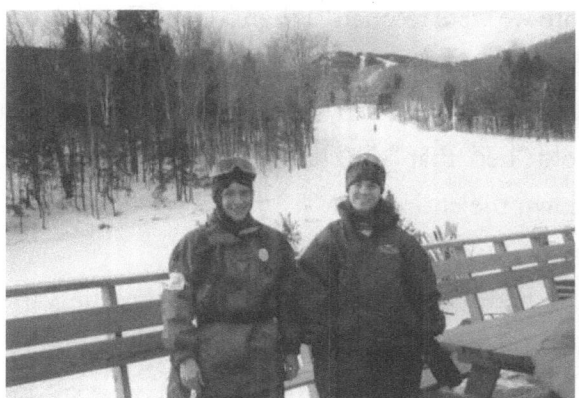

In the past, I have had the occasion to travel out of country with my parents as well as with friends. On three occasions, I have been to Cancun with Mom and Dad. The last two times, I took a friend to enjoy the experience

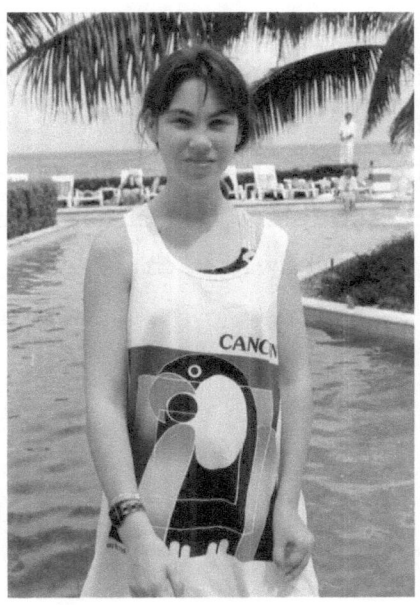

SHELLEY IN CANCUN

with me. Brian, my good friend, came along once and it proved to be a very memorable trip. Brian is gay and one of the best friends I have ever had. The night before we were to board a flight out of Boston to Cancun, Brian and I shared a room. On the morning of our flight, he called my parents' room. When my father answered, he thought it was a woman calling and immediately told "her" that "she" had the wrong room. My Dad never did live that one down the entire trip!

Brian and I had a wonderful time exploring the various night live offered in Cancun. Unfortunately, there was one evening for him when he needed a little help getting back to the room because of the partying that went on previously. Brian was always protective of me and I never worried when we were out together. The following morning's breakfast was a bit sedate for him, but that did not influence the remaining vacation time we had with one another.

I have long lost touch with him as, with most people, individuals find their own paths to take. Brian always accepted my disability without any notice given or favoritism given to me because of it. He was always one to take me by my hand, my left hand, and proudly walk with me anytime we were together. There are many things to remember him by, but this one act of kindness shown to me will always be cherished.

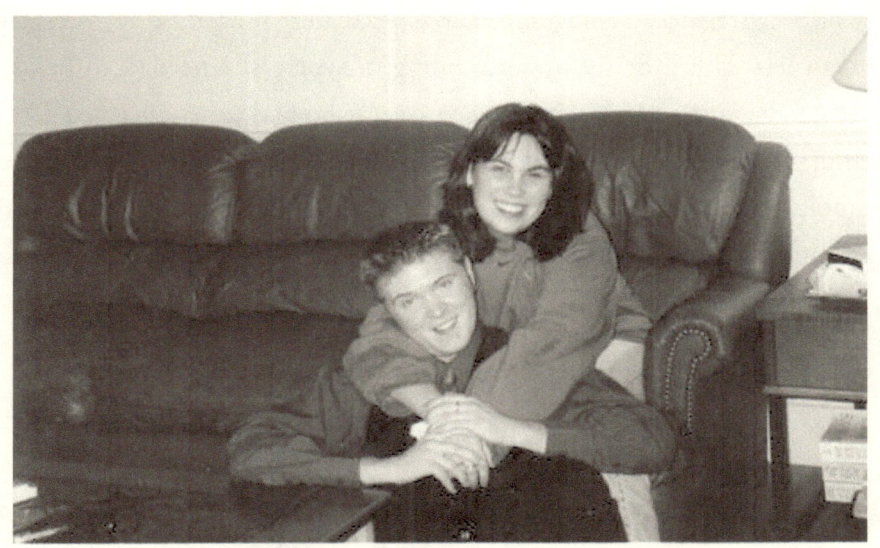

BRIAN AND SHELLEY

Kait Floberg has been another great friend to me. We have been on a couple of trips together, one also to Cancun. The other was a family cruise that Kait invited me to enjoy in the Caribbean Islands. Each time I have traveled with Kait, I have had some very memorable experiences. She has been a steady friend over the many years we have spent time together. Her family has also been tremendously kind to me.

On one particular cruise, I had the wonderful occasion to make the acquaintance of a mother of a young child who experienced like-affects of cerebral palsy as myself. This Lady sought out as much information pertaining to how I dealt with my disability as possible. She was, of course, curious as to how I dealt with my C.P. in the hope of gaining insight into how to assist her own Daughter with the youth's future quality of life.

This experience, I must admit, was extremely rewarding for me. The woman left with a better understanding of where she needed to be as a result of gleaning from someone like myself who had experienced to date a seemingly overwhelming challenge to face life with the utmost positive of outlooks. I will never forget this opportunity to dispel myths of what was to come and the hope that presented itself in dealing with future occurrences to live life to the fullest.

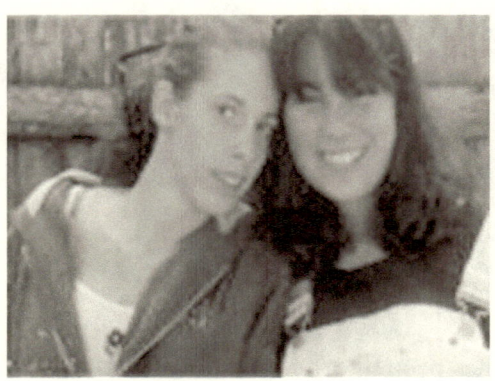

KAIT AND SHELLEY

Crystal Cranston, mentioned earlier, and I have been on trips together both in State as well as out of the country. We invited her to go on a cruise to the Western Caribbean one winter and had a great time. There is a great photo of my family and Crystal as we were negotiating Dunn's River Falls in Jamaica. On other occasions, I have enjoyed ski trips with her and her family to the Maine mountains during several winters.

My Father picked up flying again after his military retirement by renting a Schweitzer 300CBi two-seat helicopter locally. He took me with him on several flights. Each time, he let me take the cyclic and fly for an extensive period. We would fly down the coast of Maine in the summertime and enjoy the ocean scenery. During the autumn months, we would marvel at the beautiful foliage colors that looked like a patchwork quilt.

My Dad remarked that I had a great "touch" and feel for what the helicopter was going to do. As time went on, he let me fly more and more by my maintaining a certain heading and altitude. It was a great experience for me. I never would have enjoyed this type of accomplishment with any other pilot, or even by myself due to my pre-existing physical conditions.

My Father's severe and hard landing one October morning caused his helicopter days to end after logging over 2,200 flight hours. It was fortunate that both he and his passenger were not injured in the mishap. This occurrence was a devastating blow to my Father. He has never gotten over what the FAA deemed as pilot error.

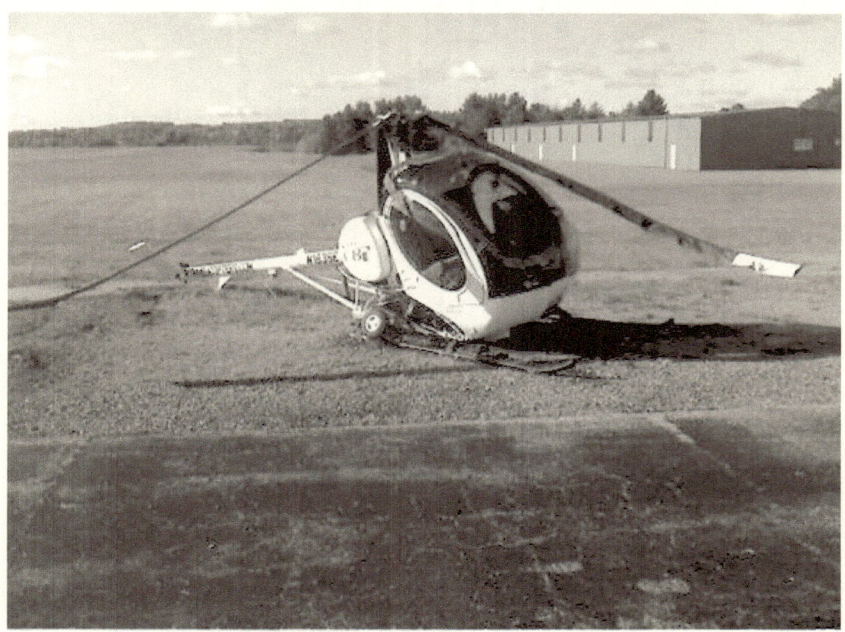

MY FATHER'S HELICOPTER MISHAP

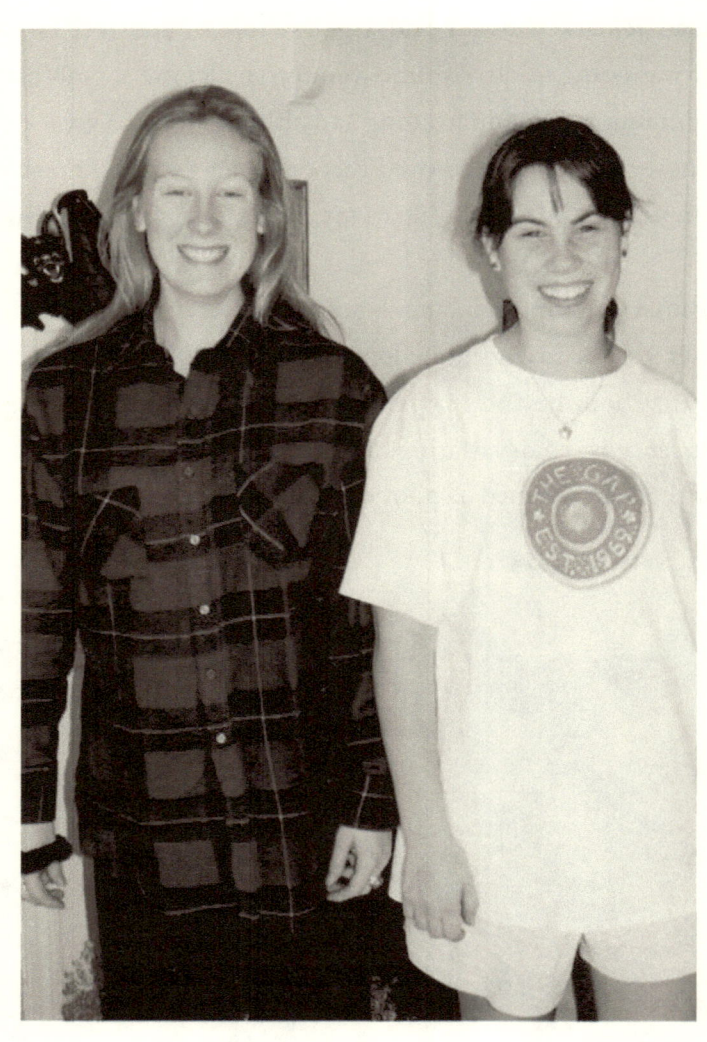

CRYSTAL AND SHELLEY

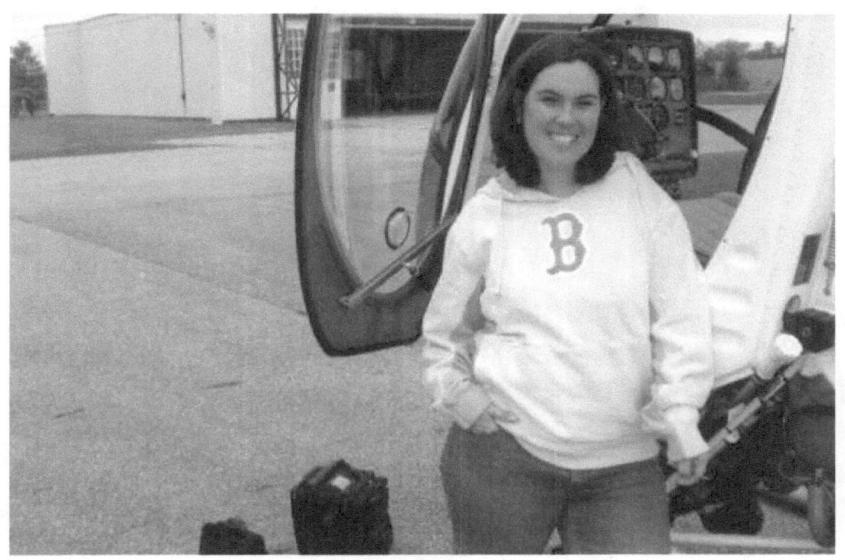

SHELLEY STANDING BY THE SCHWEITZER 300 CBi

EPILOGUE

S INCE WRITING MY story to date on paper, I have continued to work with the physically-disadvantaged at the Morrison Center. The joy that I experience daily is immeasurable. Naturally, there are days that present varying degrees of challenges. I try to meet each and every one as an experience from which to learn.

I am also hopeful that, one day, science will arrive to the point where a better understanding of what may be available to further curb, if not eliminate seizure disorders. There are many knowledgeable field researchers who continue to do extraordinary work in seeking solutions to help those of us who have the hope to live without fear or anxiety of experiencing this mind-numbing occurrence. And hope is sometimes all we have to latch onto.

I wish to thank my Parents for helping me put this work together. They both have been wonderful in assisting me to capture my life in this recounting of what it is like to live my life as a normal physically-disadvantaged youth and young adult. Thank you, Mom and Dad! You will always continue to be my Champions!